# Praise for *Bo*

"Erica Hornthal is a longtime force as an advocate for the full recognition of movement practices into mainstream psychotherapy. As an inclusive ambassador for the healing power of dance and movement, she brings her vast experience into print form with *Body Aware*. I truly believe that everyone wanting to befriend or deepen their relationship with their bodies can benefit from working with this book. Written in accessible and friendly language, it will help you to see that dance is about much more than dance, and the healing journey involves much more than working with our rational minds."

—JAMIE MARICH, PhD, LPCC-S, LICDC-CS, REAT, RYT-500, founder of the Institute for Creative Mindfulness and author of *Trauma and the 12 Steps*

"Erica Hornthal, in this groundbreaking book, helps us appreciate the intersection of these insights: that changing the activity of the body facilitates larger personal changes. With an engaging blend of research, case studies, and practical exercises, she demonstrates that change can occur from bottom-up, and not only from top-down. For practicing mental health practitioners and their clients, this is a game-changer."

—BRETT N. STEENBARGER, PhD, teaching professor of psychiatry and behavioral sciences, SUNY Upstate Medical University

"Erica's dance therapy brings peace and joy to your heart."

—MARC WEISSBLUTH, MD, Professor Emeritus of Clinical Pediatrics, Feinberg School of Medicine, Northwestern University

"Erica Hornthal brilliantly illustrates that showing up in this life begins by Simply Be-ing in our bodies."

—JESSICA ZWEIG, CEO of SimplyBe agency and best-selling author

"Erica brings a deep knowledge of how we can better listen to what our own bodies are trying to tell us—and how movement can change how we feel and experience the world."

—JENNIFER STAHL, content director for DanceMedia and editor in chief of *Dance* magazine

"Hornthal has written an incredibly thoughtful and wonderfully poignant book that is both refreshingly insightful and extremely practical. Full of action-based exercises and scientifically informed strategies for healing both the most subtle and most prominent of emotional scars, *Body Aware* is a must-read for anyone looking to deepen their understanding of just how strongly linked our minds and bodies are. A fascinating read from cover to cover."

—HELAINA HOVITZ REGAL, journalist and author of *After 9/11*

"*Body Aware* is just the prescription you need to reset your body's state of alarm, resolve emotional and physical 'dis-ease,' and cultivate and maintain the healthy synergy between your body and mind."

—DR. RUSSELL KENNEDY, THE ANXIETY MD, author of *The Anxiety Rx*

"Pick up *Body Aware* and find a new best friend, your own wild and wonderful moving self. Erica brings what is elusive to most—the power of moving with awareness—into all aspects of your life. You'll feel enriched, encouraged, and gently challenged to expand your vitality and creativity with powerfully simple practices and shifts that bridge mind and body with new moves."

—KATHLYN HENDRICKS, PhD, BC-DMT, best-selling author of *Conscious Loving*

"Erica Hornthal, in her book *Body Aware*, has pointed us toward a fundamental truth—that movement forms the basis for change, well-being, and growth. Because movement permeates everything we do and are, it can help us not only physically, but also mentally, socially, and emotionally. Hornthal importantly shows us how to challenge our entrenched habits of being and doing through movement, seeing it as a catalyst for liberation from that which is entrenched within us. This book does not proscribe certain movements—it assists us in finding certain movements within us and leveraging them for our and the world's transformation. Well done!"

"*Body Aware* presents a unique perspective—from that of a dance/movement therapist—on the power of movement to enhance mental health and emotional resilience. Blending examples from her work with clients with a lively mosaic of options for personal practice, Erica Hornthal guides you through an introduction to befriending your body, and thus yourself, at a deeper level. With the many outer distractions of our multimedia world, this call inward provides a timely remedy for the soul."

"Erica places the body front and center in *Body Aware,* an ode to health and healing. Having gone on my own ride with my body as a gymnast, professional ballet dancer, and now body-language expert, I appreciate that Erica captures the power and imperative we all face by shining a light on what our bodies have to say. For anyone who feels their body has been relegated to the shadows and neglected, this book is a must-read."

"*Body Aware* is a brilliant, compassionate, thoroughly researched, deeply important book. If you have a body, I highly recommend you read it!"

"*Body Aware* intuitively reconnects you to the most important parts of yourself through the body. A treasure of knowledge and exploration awaits you every step of the way."

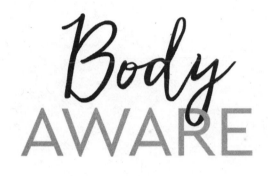

Body
AWARE

# *Body* AWARE

### Rediscover Your Mind-Body Connection, Stop Feeling Stuck, and Improve Your Mental Health through Simple Movement Practices

## ERICA HORNTHAL, LCPC, BC-DMT

### FOREWORD BY NICOLE LEPERA, PHD
#### THE HOLISTIC PSYCHOLOGIST
#### BEST-SELLING AUTHOR OF *HOW TO DO THE WORK*

North Atlantic Books
Huichin, unceded Ohlone land
*aka* Berkeley, California

Published by                                   Cover art © Dollariz/Shutterstock.com
North Atlantic Books                           Book design by Happenstance-Type-O-Rama
Huichin, unceded Ohlone land                   Cover design by Mimi Bark
*aka* Berkeley, California

Printed in Canada

*Body Aware* is sponsored and published by North Atlantic Books, an educational nonprofit based in the unceded Ohlone land Huichin (*aka* Berkeley, CA) that collaborates with partners to develop cross-cultural perspectives, nurture holistic views of art, science, the humanities, and healing, and seed personal and global transformation by publishing work on the relationship of body, spirit, and nature.

North Atlantic Books' publications are distributed to the US trade and internationally by Penguin Random House Publisher Services. For further information, visit our website at www.northatlanticbooks.com.

MEDICAL DISCLAIMER: The following information is intended for general information purposes only. Individuals should always see their health care provider before administering any suggestions made in this book. Any application of the material set forth in the following pages is at the reader's discretion and is their sole responsibility.

Library of Congress Cataloging-in-Publication Data

Names: Hornthal, Erica, 1983- author.
Title: Body aware : rediscover your mind-body connection, stop feeling
    stuck, and improve your mental health with simple movement practices /
    by Erica Hornthal, LCPC, BC-DMT ; foreword by Dr. Nicole LePera.
Description: Berkeley, California : North Atlantic Books, 2022. | Includes
    bibliographical references and index.
Identifiers: LCCN 2021059172 (print) | LCCN 2021059173 (ebook) | ISBN
    9781623176891 (trade paperback) | ISBN 9781623176907 (ebook)
Subjects: LCSH: Mind and body. | Emotions. | Awareness. | Movement,
    Psychology of.
Classification: LCC BF161 .H767 2022  (print) | LCC BF161 (ebook) | DDC
    128/.2—dc23/eng/20220322
LC record available at https://lccn.loc.gov/2021059172
LC ebook record available at https://lccn.loc.gov/2021059173

1 2 3 4 5 6 7 8 9 MARQUIS 27 26 25 24 23 22

This book includes recycled material and material from well-managed forests. North Atlantic Books is committed to the protection of our environment. We print on recycled paper whenever possible and partner with printers who strive to use environmentally responsible practices.

To my clients, who taught me
that just because someone cannot speak
doesn't mean they have nothing to say.

# Contents

# Preface

This is not just another book about exercise, meditation, yoga, or embodiment and it's not written by a neuroscientist, a professor, a biomechanist, or even a dance psychologist. The entire book is written from my perspective and experience as a student, client, and practitioner of Westernized dance/movement therapy. While dance as a healing modality has been around for millennia, this book explores methodologies and techniques from my own education and practice in this field. As a passionate practitioner and advocate for dance/movement therapy, I believe our work has been overlooked for far too long.

Dance/movement therapy in its Westernized form has been a professional field since around the 1950s, but on a grander scale few people outside of the field are familiar with the modality. Dance/movement therapy is a form of psychotherapy that focuses on the mind-body connection; putting the body in the driver's seat rather than relying solely on the mind. The methods and techniques that have been passed down are still questioned by modern medicine and minimized by many "authority figures" in mental health who label it as adjunct and alternative. I advocate for this work for the people who came before me and have put their entire being into educating and sharing the wonder and sheer magic that unfolds when witnessing a person claiming their space in this world by showing up in their body. In writing this book, I pay tribute to future students and therapists, not to mention the clients who, despite debilitating illnesses, childhood trauma, and unbelievable loss and grief, choose to show up in this life through movement.

It feels necessary to acknowledge that since this book is written from my perspective—that of a white Jewish cisgender woman—I know I do

not speak for everyone and I understand that even my own body awareness and view of the work comes from a privileged Eurocentric lens.
Even more reason to highlight that this book is not meant as a universal
remedy, but as a guide for anyone reading to claim their own experiences
and how each experience is individually embodied.

To read and gain from this book, you are not required to have any previous knowledge or understanding of somatics or other body-centered
practices. This book will provide you with accessible and digestible ideas,
tips, and resources on the link between how you move and your mental
health. In my opinion, most nonacademic books have skirted around just
how much movement influences mental health.

Furthermore, this focus on movement is not about exercising, but
recognizing your own relationship to movement, exploring your current movement habits, and expanding your own range of and capacity
for movement so you can improve your mental health and create a life
full of meaning and purpose. This book aims to show you how your
movements—especially the ones that you aren't even aware of—shape
your interactions, relationships, and behaviors.

Before you start reading, I want to introduce some important terms
and ideas that are central to this book. The term *body* includes the top
of the head to the bottom of the feet, not just from the neck down. I also
want to make clear that while definitions and principles discussed in this
book will be cited in literature and resources, I acknowledge that their
origins go well beyond these references. A fellow dance/movement therapist, Neha Christopher, pointed out that there is a difference between
"Western nomenclature and Western invention."[1]

While the references may point to Western invention, it is important
to know that that is more often a product of Western civilization rein-
venting and taking ownership of customs and traditions originated by
other cultures. I will do my best to pay honor and homage to the cultural
origins of these practices and acknowledge that the work I do is possible
because of the healers, body workers, and ancestors who came before me.

*Body Aware* is a guidebook that addresses how the way you move
impacts who you are. Embracing this approach is about more than

adopting an exercise routine or a meditation practice; it comes down to the following:

- Identifying where you hold your emotions in your body
- Interpreting your body's unique language
- Listening to and recognizing bodily sensations in order to identify emotional blockages
- Exploring how the smallest involuntary movements play a vital role in how you function
- Expanding your movement vocabulary to enhance your resilience and manage your emotions amid life's greatest challenges

It's time to redefine what movement is and how it plays a role in your life, so you can harness the power of your movement to step into your greatest potential and start creating the life you want by changing the way you *move* through it.

# Foreword

As a holistic psychologist who's been closely tied to Erica Hornthal's work, I know the importance of a mind-body approach to wellness. In *Body Aware* Erica takes a revolutionary approach to improve mental health and to help people stop feeling stuck. Today's mental health system doesn't fully take into account how important the body is, and this book represents a long-overdue paradigm shift in the way we think of treating mental health issues. In my experience, without bringing the body into mental health treatment we do a disservice to both the clients and practitioners. I am asked consistently by therapists, "How can I bring the body into treatment?" and this book answers that much-needed call. As more and more practitioners become aware of the mind-body connection, this book will only become more important and relevant. Erica's delivery is relatable, comprehensive, and straightforward. It's filled with compassion and curiosity, two things that are foundational in healing.

Erica understands that the body, and specifically movement, allows us to have access to heal the mind. *Body Aware* gives the reader practical and tangible tools to become more aware of our bodies. Today, so many of us are suffering from depression, anxious or racing thoughts, or the inability to feel connected to the people we love. Many of us have learned to cope with life through leaving our body. We dissociate because we are overwhelmed with the present moment. Using our intentional movement in safe ways allows us to return to the body. As we return to the body, our mental health changes. We are more present, our thoughts are more calm and peaceful, and we are more able to express ourselves creatively. Everyone wants to be more fulfilled, happy, and at peace. *Body Aware* provides a clear roadmap for how to create this in your own life. It's the hopeful medicine needed at a time in our world where there's so much fear and unpredictability.

Through this book, I learned more about where I hold my own emotions and how to have a different relationship with the sensations of my body. It's clear that Erica has a gift in presenting this information in a way that everyone can learn something new, and more importantly everyone can actually integrate. I also found it to be incredibly inclusive, offering tips for people who are disabled or limited in their ability to move. This matters, because so often we have an image of movement for a select group of people. In *Body Aware,* there is a space for everyone, which reshapes the often intimidating space of bodywork.

I, like Erica, believe that you can change your life and your thoughts through intentional movement. I'm thrilled for the reader who will have a new relationship with their body, and the way they see the world. If you're looking to heal, this is the book for you. If you're looking to use bodywork within your own practice, this book is for you. As a psychologist, educator, and author, I recommend this book to everyone wanting to learn more about emotions, movement, and human behavior.

—NICOLE LEPERA, PhD,
The Holistic Psychologist and
best-selling author of *How to Do the Work*, 2022

# Part 1

# EXPLORING
# HOW YOU MOVE

# INTRODUCTION
## Your Movement Matters

*Nothing is more revealing than movement.*
—MARTHA GRAHAM

## My Journey

I began dancing at a young age. You may know the story yourself. Kid dances all over the house. Mom puts kid in a formal dance class. Kid is happy! I can remember trying other hobbies and sports only to find myself back in the dance studio. I always loved to dance, but it wasn't until my family was relocated from Tampa, Florida, to the North Shore of Chicago, Illinois, that dance became so much more to me than an art form or hobby. In fact, I didn't realize just how much I needed dance until it was not readily available or accessible.

While there were benefits to this move, it was a huge adjustment—to say the least. At fifteen, moving away from family, friends, and a community that shaped my identity was only exacerbated when I became what felt like no more than a number in a high school that prided itself on excellence and competition. If you are familiar with the 2004 film *Mean Girls,* you have a "Hollywoodized" idea of what I experienced. While my particular circumstance was not identical to the main character, much like her I did struggle to find my way and experienced an existential crisis when all the things I knew to be true about myself were questioned. I naturally turned to dance, but even that was met with barriers.

Transferring to a new school and community made for a rough transition as I attempted to navigate and integrate into established programs with auditions and assessments already underway.

With time and after a lot of tears, I slowly found my footing, and ultimately made my way back to the dance studio. Dance, more than anything, became an outlet, a coping mechanism, and a lifeline. I didn't dance to fit in or be popular. I danced because it was familiar, stable, and reliable. It was a way to come home and belong to myself when I didn't know where I belonged in the world—let alone my community.

Long before I knew about the field of dance/movement therapy, dance inherently became my therapy. I may not have realized it at the time, but I needed it to get through challenging transitions in my life. When I think back on those transitions—whether it was relocating with my family, discovering my identity during adolescence, on the cusp of exploring my independence as a college freshman amid the challenges and fears directly following 9/11, or navigating the COVID-19 pandemic—I realize now that those experiences constricted my emotional expression by restricting my physical movements.

Pain and discomfort create constriction in the body. The more restriction present in the body, the more confined we become in our minds. Without my realizing it, dance kept me from playing small, or limiting my presence, even when life experience and the world had other plans. Learning breathing techniques through Pilates during my high school dance class created core support, which reinforced psychological constructs of identity. Experiencing some aspects of West African dance during my freshman year in college kept me grounded and connected to the Earth, which for me facilitated a sense of internal safety and connectedness. And through taking up ballroom dance, not only did I learn to communicate my needs and trust in a partner, but also I embodied emotional resilience learning to transition from the elongated steps of the waltz to the intricate sharp steps of the tango.

These are just a few examples of how moving my body in new, unexpected, and often challenging ways allowed me to counterbalance the effects of life. Through movement I discovered that I was resourceful,

4

creative, resilient, motivated, and strong—physically and mentally. Furthermore, I was able to authentically maneuver my psychological landscape by finding my own way around the dance floor.

It is my hope that my use of movement as a catalyst for change and acceptance shows that it is possible for anyone. This is because it isn't about the "right way" but rather "your way" of recognizing the innate healing power of movement with regard to your individual culture, gender, race, or religion and how it supports your own personal mental health. Whether you are faced with egregious oppression, political unrest, a traumatic childhood, a life-changing diagnosis, debilitating anxiety, or the developmental challenges of adolescence, the body is a carrier for all experiences. As this book will explore, dancing through difficult times literally taught me to keep *moving through* my life—and how I moved played a huge role in how I coped, managed, and operated *in* the world.

Realizing that dance and mental health as professions were not mutually exclusive, I decided to explore career paths in dance and psychology, ultimately finding my way to the field of dance/movement therapy in the hopes of using movement in a clinical setting to improve mental health for individuals needing a holistic approach. I ultimately attended graduate school for dance/movement therapy and counseling.

Dance/movement therapy, often referred to as dance therapy, is not just a phrase or a hashtag. According to the American Dance Therapy Association (ADTA), "Dance/movement therapy is the psychotherapeutic use of movement to promote emotional, social, cognitive and physical integration of the individual."[2] Dr. Jennifer Frank Tantia, dance/movement therapist and somatic psychotherapist, states, "It is a psychotherapeutic process that creates balance in the nervous system, ownership of one's own body, and agency through movement. . . ."[3]

Despite the name, dance/movement therapy is not only about dance. While it places an emphasis on dance, it is more about the use of movement and the body's language as an inherent form of expression. As mentioned in the *New York Times* best seller *Maybe You Should Talk to Someone*, with regard to her own experience of dance in healing, author Lori Gottlieb says, "When we dance, we express our buried feelings, talking through our bodies instead of our minds."[4] A participant is not required to be a dancer, have any previous dance experience, or any coordination for that matter. Dance therapists don't teach people to become better dancers, but rather support clients to connect to the innate mover inside. Even becoming a dance therapist doesn't require that the practitioner be a seasoned professional dancer, but that they have the ability to access different movement characteristics and the capacity to use their body as a vessel for empathic connection in the therapeutic relationship. It is about using movement—a core component of dance—to express the innermost thoughts, desires, and needs of the individual, uncovering what is too deep to express through words alone.

While dance/movement therapy is not the only option out there, it feels like a secret that I want to shout from the rooftops. In my opinion, dance/movement therapy is the most comprehensive form of psychotherapy that most people have never heard of. As a talk therapist would practice reflective listening, dance/movement therapists practice *embodied* listening. Dance/movement therapists do not just listen with their ears. They listen with their entire bodies. We can reflect what we see in the body's language and tone of the client, as you would in a mirror. Kinesthetic empathy[5] and attunement create connection, trust, and communication on another level. Dr. Danielle Fraenkel, dance/movement therapist and educator, says, "Kinesthetic empathy is the keystone of dance/movement therapy; the pivotal guide to building trusting therapeutic relationships with our clients."[6] Imagine you are in the middle of nowhere and desperately trying to get anything but static on your car's radio. Attunement can be seen as the act of the therapist finely tuning their body to match the client's radio frequency. This further illustrates the immense validation and satisfaction both can encounter when the static becomes audible recognizable sound.

Dance/movement at its core becomes the catalyst and vessel for communication, trust, and relationship. Additionally, dance/movement becomes the means for observation, assessment, and intervention in addition to the use of verbal processing. It is essential that the client integrates both as we are tending to the mind-body connection and bringing the body into a symbiotic relationship with the mind. Dance/movement therapy supports the creation of a symbiotic relationship between the body, mind, and spirit.

For the past decade, I've worked with clients from ages three to 107 from all different backgrounds, using movement through the lens of dance/movement therapy to address concerns like anxiety, chronic pain, depression, and cognitive and developmental differences, such as Alzheimer's disease, traumatic brain injury, and autism. Through this work I began to see a common thread with my clients. The inability to connect to the body's innate wisdom and knowledge was gravely impacting quality of life. Becoming known as "The Therapist Who Moves You," I found myself literally helping my clients *move* out of their own ways and *move* into lives of purpose, passion, connection, expression, and meaning.

In graduate school and even in my early years of being a professional, I didn't realize the extent to which dance and movement could support healing. I knew how it made me feel and that I could use dance and movement to convey feelings, but to get out of my head and listen to my body was a whole other world. Honestly, it is a world I am still navigating and will continue to discover. When you have been wired to live in your mind it is both scary and liberating to think, challenge, and explore what lives in your body. When you feel imprisoned by your mind, your body can be what sets you free.

My practice as a dance/movement therapist has allowed me to expand my own movement vocabulary (an embodied dictionary of sorts) and my own body knowledge, which supports my identity, my core belief system, and my values. It serves as a compass that guides me back home when I feel lost. Dance was an outlet, but it has become so much more. This is the basis for this book. I have seen firsthand how people get in their own way of achieving their potential by limiting their movement. People play small and limit their presence in their bodies, and while this is often designed to create a sense of safety, this unconsciously spills over to other areas like relationships, jobs, even everyday interactions.

If you want to show up in this life, you've got to begin by showing up in your body. That means examining and deconstructing *how* you show up in your body and understanding that how you *currently* live in your body is not the only way. If you want to change facets of your life, begin by observing how your body currently moves and what happens in response to those changes.

*Body Aware* will allow you to explore this. All you have to do is become curious about how your movement impacts who you are, and bring awareness to how you move. You do not have to be a dancer, enjoy dance, or take any dance classes to reap the full benefits of this book. In fact, a bulk of the work I have done in my private practice has been with individuals who are either chair bound or at times bed bound. These are individuals living with degenerative diseases like Alzheimer's, movement disorders like Parkinson's, or even people born with traumatic brain injuries or developmental differences. No matter how small or inaccessible someone's movement may appear, the potential for expansion and connection through the body is always possible. Every human body tells a story, and as you begin to understand, dance and movement in general is another way of telling that story as well as rewriting the narrative. You are moving all the time, and it is about time that you harnessed the power of your movement to face challenges, overcome adversity, and achieve your greatest dreams.

## Challenging the Status Quo

When you think of change and the body, you may think of diet and exercise, but that is not what I am talking about. Yes, change begins in the body—but not by altering its aesthetics. Dr. Peter Lovatt, English dance psychologist and author of *The Dance Cure,* writes, "If you want to make changes to the way you think, then start with the way you move your body."[7] Challenging your body's status quo can allow you to move out of your comfort zone and eventually embrace new movement possibilities. This is how lasting change occurs and where I believe the quest for personal growth begins.

Awareness is the key to change. We cannot change anything if we lack awareness that something is out of balance or misaligned. Many of us are so resigned to living a life of status quo that we don't challenge or question the need for change. Furthermore, we lack the initiative to take responsibility for our own circumstances. We are perfectly comfortable living in a world we have created that makes us prisoners to stress, burnout, apathy, and overwhelming anxiety. In fact, that is often worn as a badge of honor. The amount of stress endured in a job is often a sign of accomplishment. This line from the 2006 film, *The Devil Wears Prada,* illustrates this point. Nigel (Stanley Tucci) says to Andrea (Anne Hathaway), "Let me know when your entire life goes up in smoke, then it's time for a promotion."[8] This is the mantra for so much of corporate life.

We tell ourselves that it will change when we get that promotion, once the kids are "out of that phase," when we retire, or when we get through the next however many days, months, or even years. We idolize a celebrity culture and binge-watch "reality" television, which is anything but real, to escape our own hectic reality. We distract ourselves with technology to lessen the suffering that comes from space and quiet, because it is in the downtime that our true thoughts emerge. Some of us believe we need to go on expensive retreats in remote tropical destinations to get back in touch with ourselves so that we can go back to tolerating the everyday grind.

Why is it that we go through life never challenging the status quo? We make excuses for our situations, reason our way out of wanting more for ourselves, and minimize our dissatisfaction with our lives. We may even convince ourselves that we are happy, or worse, convince ourselves that we are undeserving and therefore happiness is overrated and unattainable.

Challenging ourselves can be uncomfortable and painful, which is one big reason we opt out of it. We might feel like we have no power over our circumstances. What happens to us may not be in our control, but we *can* control how we respond to those circumstances and the behaviors we exhibit. The less we take responsibility for our actions, the more we perpetuate our lack of power and our helplessness in our situation. Another reason we overlook change is because we like comfort. As long as we remain in a predictable environment, no matter how stress-provoking it may be, it is still not as bad as being uncomfortable. We have adjusted and evolved to our environment so much that we would rather sacrifice our emotional health than sit in discomfort and feel everything that comes with it. Lastly, it is really hard work. Recognizing that we are not living up to our potential can be painful, and making the changes necessary to realize that potential is not the easy path—but then again, nothing worth having comes easily.

I have seen many clients in my practice who know that something needs to change, yet do not act on that potential so they can cling to the familiarity of comfort and illusion of stability. Instead of connecting to the body and processing our issues, so many of us buffer; we consume, we scroll, we complain, we turn into couch potatoes. If we think of movement as exercise, it becomes one more thing to do in an overly packed schedule and we are less likely to do it.

Here's a little secret. You do not have to sacrifice your potential for comfort. Read that again and notice how your body receives that information. When you choose to remain comfortable, you do yourself a disservice by limiting your own ability to achieve. You emotionally and physically hold yourself back from opportunities related to personal growth, occupation, relationships, and even love. However, the answer doesn't lie in jumping into the deep end. The answer lies within your body and the ability to notice the discomfort while learning to manage it simultaneously. It is in the emotional discomfort that we can increase our awareness of how this impacts the body and therefore the mind.

Through the body you can learn to confront, maybe even embrace discomfort by exposing yourself to it. You can release the stress, the burnout, the overwhelming anxiety, but it is going to be uncomfortable at first and won't be easy. But again, change is not about being comfortable. It is about learning to identify and sit in discomfort.

You may ask, "Why fix something if it isn't broken?" That is the problem! We often lack the awareness that something is broken, because we are too cushioned by our comfortable bubbles. To be clear, we as individuals are not broken. What's broken is the system—a system that devalues mental health, self-care, and the need for balance. You have the ability to change the status quo, to thrive—not just survive—and to live a life of meaning and purpose no matter what your emotional and physical circumstances may be.

If awareness is the key to change, then movement is the catalyst for awareness. English writer and philosopher Aldous Huxley wrote, "Consciousness is only possible through change, change is only possible through movement."[9] Your greatest tool and most underutilized resource to bring awareness and implement change is your body. Bessel van der Kolk, author of *The Body Keeps the Score,* says that for change to occur, "People need to become aware of their sensations and the way that their bodies interact with the world around them."[10] It starts with challenging the way you move. Once you begin challenging how you move, you will naturally begin to expand your movement repertoire—the stock of movements you have at your disposal.

## Challenging the Way You Move

Just because you have spent most of your life moving a certain way doesn't mean that it has to stay that way. The good news is that you are already moving all the time. Even when sedentary, your heart is beating, your lungs are expanding, and your eyes are blinking. This is not something that needs to be taught, but rather a new awareness you can gain that will wake up a greater potential. When you move the "right way" for *you,* the body becomes the tool and catalyst for that untapped and unrealized potential. When you add to your current movement vocabulary, you open yourself up to opportunities and expand your horizons through meaningful connection to yourself, to others, and to the world.

Try this. Sit in your chair with your chin lowered, eyes down, and torso slouched. Ask yourself, "If I stayed in this position for an extended period of time, how might this impact my mood?" Now consider what posture you take on when you are looking at your phone. How often do you engage with a screen? These interactions influence how you move, which directly impacts how you feel. We know that posture impacts mood,[11] but did you know that you can learn to move your body in new ways to promote a healthier mood?

In essence, you can change the way your brain is wired—and thereby create meaningful relationships and find purpose—by changing your body's habitual movement patterns. How you move or don't move is directly correlated to your mental health.[12] Results from a 2017 study showed that body posture impacts regulation of emotion. In particular, the study demonstrated "for the first time that negative mood is not just associated with a stooped body posture, stooped body posture also resulted in relatively less negative mood regulation."[13] In a study conducted in 2019, researchers found correlations between the mental status of walkers with regard to anxiety and depression and their natural gait.[14] While more research needs to be conducted, I have seen firsthand with my clients a connection between intensity of thoughts and speed of movement. Intentionally slowing down our movements can facilitate slowing down our thought patterns and as a result manage our stress and anxiety. The *way* we move impacts what we think and feel, for better or worse.

One way I challenge my movement on a regular basis is by using my nondominant hand. While I do not recommend signing important documents or checks with your nondominant hand, I encourage you to doodle with it. Use your nondominant hand to brush your teeth or hair. Hold your Starbucks with it. Try putting your pants on the other leg first. Change the way you cross your legs, arms, and even fingers. This not only changes your movement patterns, but actually creates new neural connections and rewires your brain for change. When your brain becomes more pliable, you increase your tolerance to everyday stressors, which allows you to cope with a range of emotions.

But it doesn't stop there. This book is going to teach you not only how to move, but also why moving in new ways can enhance your life, ease stress, and reshape and rewire your brain. To make lasting changes, you must integrate new movement "words" into your body's dictionary through daily practice. Much as you would practice a new skill to truly embrace it and hone your newfound ability, the same must happen with regard to movement in order to make these new movements part of your everyday life.

By harnessing your natural ability to communicate through the body and listen to what your body is trying to tell you, you can restore balance, become more emotionally resilient, and realize your greatest potential. Given the proper tools, your body will literally set you free.

## Breaking It Down

*Body Aware* is conveniently broken down into three parts:

- Exploring How You Move
- Movement Is a Catalyst for Change
- Transformation through Movement

In the part "Exploring How You Move," you will explore your individual connection to movement: how it is defined and how you can redefine it to increase your awareness and potential through movement. This part lays the foundation and groundwork for becoming more aware of your body.

"Movement Is a Catalyst for Change" will break down the way certain movements influence emotions, thoughts, and feelings—which often correlate to how you relate to yourself, others, and the environment. You will gain an understanding of how movement can create change in areas like relationships, career, and connection to Self.

Lastly, "Transformation through Movement" is about honoring all the ways movement supports lasting change. You will explore how movement supports resilience and how it encourages acceptance of differing abilities. This part also provides hands-on exercises and real-life case examples, leaving you empowered and confident that change for the better is possible and can be permanent.

Within each chapter, you can expect mini-exercises designed as breaks to increase awareness and presence so that the information can be integrated and put into practice. Chapters are full of composite cases, rather than case studies, to protect the identities of clients. Each chapter ends with "Movement Prescriptions" and takeaways designed to highlight key talking points that will inspire you to deepen your own work and continue the conversation.

This book is not just another "how-to" guide. It is a *lifestyle change*. It is a real contribution to all of us who are drowning in distraction. When you challenge how you take up space in your life, you have the ability to show up in ways you never imagined. Not sure how you can make a difference? Start with your own body. Change the way you move and permanently change your body, your mood, and your outlook on life. It's time to explore what it means to be aware—physically and emotionally. It's time to redefine what movement is and how it plays a role in your life so you can harness the power of your movement to step into your greatest potential and start creating the life you want by changing the way you move through it.

Are you ready to *move*?

## TAKEAWAYS

* Dance/movement therapy supports the creation of a symbiotic relationship between body, mind, and spirit.

* When you have been wired to live in your mind, it is both scary and liberating to think, challenge, and explore what lives in your body.

* If you want to change facets of your life, begin by observing how your body moves in response to those changes.

* You do not have to sacrifice your potential for comfort.

* If awareness is the key to change, then movement is the catalyst for awareness.

# 1

# BECOMING BODY AWARE

*Awareness is like the sun.*
*When it shines on things, they are transformed.*
—THICH NHAT HANH

## Bringing Awareness to the Self

How *aware* are you right now? Let's explore.

I invite you to draw your attention to the movements you are engaging in as you read this book. Focus on your posture, how you are sitting or reclining as you read. Notice how your body is shaped by the object you are resting on. Are you comfortable? Do you notice any areas of tension or discomfort in the way you are sitting? Now take an inventory of what parts of your body are touching the surface on which you are resting. Notice what parts of your body are touching other body parts. Are your feet touching the ground or elevated? Pay attention to how you are holding or listening to this book. Are your hands clenched? Notice how your eyes glance over the words. Notice the internal involuntary movements that are occurring in your body. Draw focus to your breath, heartbeat, even your eyes as they blink.

Now think back to when you woke up this morning. How did you wake up? Were you startled by an alarm clock? Did you naturally wake up as the sun shone through your window? Perhaps a family member or pet woke you up by jumping on you. However you woke up, what was the first movement you remember engaging in? Perhaps you intensely rubbed your eyes, slowly yawned, indulgently stretched, abruptly turned off the alarm clock, or haphazardly reached for your cell phone on your nightstand. Consider how you got out of bed and all the movements you did as you got ready to start your day. Did you take your time or did you feel rushed? Were you aware or in a daze? Did you stumble and clumsily bump into things or pay attention to your surroundings as you carefully tiptoed or shuffled to the bathroom?

Up until this moment, perhaps you were aware of your workload or a deadline. You may have been aware of the time or how much or little you have of it between responsibilities and commitments. You may even be aware of that nagging headache or stuffy nose that just won't let you be, but were you aware of your emotions? More so, were you aware of the way your body was *holding* those emotions?

How you feel and how your body moves could mean the difference between surviving and thriving. Said another way . . . I believe that *how* you move impacts *who* you are and *how* you feel.

## What's Awareness Got to Do with It?

Keep in mind that so much of what we encounter on a daily basis never becomes conscious information; however, that doesn't mean that it doesn't impact us. Our bodies are receiving information all the time, and even if it doesn't get to our conscious awareness, the information is felt and sensed by the body. Information must be transferred to conscious perception in order for us to be consciously aware. This begs the question: What does it mean to be aware? Before we can dive into what it means to be *aware,* let's look at what it means to be *unaware.*

To be *unaware* means to have no knowledge of a situation or circumstance. It is synonymous to being ignorant, inattentive, unresponsive, and unconscious. While it is difficult and often unnecessary to be aware of everything all the time, I believe we are always aware of something. I began to wonder which is easier: being aware or being unaware. The more I thought about it, the clearer it became to me that it is determined by our capacity to manage the emotions that arise in the state of awareness. For myself, I actually find it harder to be unaware as I have spent countless hours studying psychotherapy and being in therapy myself. I enjoy the challenge of being aware and have put what I preach into practice. But when I am stressed or in survival mode, my scope of awareness narrows.

For someone living with an eating disorder, a history of abuse, or a traumatic childhood, being unaware may not be easy, but it may be necessary. I believe we become conditioned to being unaware in order to ease our pain. We intentionally distract ourselves so we don't have to acknowledge the messy uncomfortable feelings below the surface. The irony is that while we think we are avoiding pain and discomfort, we are actually causing ourselves more stress and unnecessary suffering. We are depleting our energy due to emotional and physical overwhelm that is only exacerbated when we bottle up those feelings, repress them, or altogether deny their existence. Research shows that in order to release trauma, we must turn to the body to repattern and rewire the nervous system. Healing must happen not just on an emotional level but on a physical one as well.[1] Additionally, recovery from trauma specifically is not possible until there is a familiarity with bodily sensations. To safely reexamine the past we must first learn to withstand and observe our physical responses.[2] As the neuroscientist Antonio Damasio highlighted, the root of self-awareness depends on physical sensations as they communicate the body's internal state of affairs.[3]

Why stop at trauma? We can use awareness of the body to rewire and repattern habits and behaviors across the board. After all, habits are an attempt at regulating the nervous system. When we feel safe we can increase and explore our ability to be present and aware. So it is vital that we foster safety and security in our bodies to allow ourselves the ability to be present and aware: mind, body, and soul.

**BODY AWARE BREAK** Take a moment to think about your personal relationship to safety. Just think of the word safety. Where do you notice it in your body? Is it present at all? Is there a movement associated with it? What qualities or characteristics does it take on? This is not a light subject, so be gentle with yourself and allow time to think about it, or if this is feeling like too much too soon, then be aware of that feeling and come back to this exercise when you are ready.

While we are very aware as infants, sensitive to the smallest environmental changes, as we grow we tend to rely less on our senses and more on our ability to logically reason why we feel a certain way. Rather than feel how emotions are manifested in the body through a clenched fist or a furrowed brow, we instead identify with thoughts. As we age, our executive functioning, a set of mental skills including working memory, flexible thinking, and self-control as well as the developing brain, seems to take over the show, unless we choose to tap into the body knowledge we already have.

I would argue that most of the world today is unaware. In fact, society has become accustomed to using devices in our daily lives that keep us in a perpetual state of unawareness. Don't get me wrong; there is a time and place for technology and many medical advances wouldn't be available without it. However, our inability to disconnect from our devices and connect to ourselves has major implications on our emotional and mental health.

Technology often impedes and limits our movement. This doesn't just mean how often we move, but also the reach of our movement or the ways in which we move through our environment. Let me introduce you to the term *kinesphere*. The Westernized concept of the *kinesphere* was shaped by Rudolf Laban. Laban defines kinesphere as "the sphere around the body whose periphery can be reached by easily extended limbs without stepping away from that place which is the point of support when standing on one foot."[4] When we engage in technology, we limit our awareness of and full use of our kinesphere or "personal space." Whether we are interacting with a computer and sitting at a desk or using a mobile device, we are limiting our range of movement, which limits our range of emotions.

It is not lost on me that technology makes movement possible for many people. Thanks to assistive technology, advances in prosthetic design, health technology, and medical advancement in general, people are moving more, better, and longer. In these specific instances, a person's kinesphere can indeed be enhanced by the use of technology.

Recent technological advancements further support the known fact that mind and body are connected. Dr. Candace Pert, author of *Molecules of Emotion,* says "recent technological innovations have allowed us to examine the molecular basis of the emotions. . . . It is the emotions, I have come to see that link mind and body."[5] The information age we are in has completely changed the way we communicate, socialize, and connect, influencing the way we move—which ultimately impacts emotional well-being. Research shows that just having a cell phone present during a conversation or meal creates enough distraction to lessen the overall satisfaction or joy with the social experience.[6] We think we can multitask, but the human brain is only designed to consciously do one task at a time. Dr. Caroline Leaf, communication pathologist and cognitive neuroscientist, says we "do busy well" because we are designed to shift quickly from one task to the next.[7] So when we attempt to multitask, things can begin to feel disjointed, chaotic, rushed, or sloppy and our attention becomes scattered.

According to James Williams, author of *Stand Out of Our Light: Freedom and Resistance in the Attention Economy,* "The new challenges we face in the Age of Attention are, on both individual and collective levels, challenges of self-regulation."[8] I could not agree more, and from a body perspective it makes total sense. Self-regulation is an embodied practice and if we are not present to the body we cannot self-regulate. Regulation of the self is dependent on the relationship you have with your body.[9]

We may be aware of the latest trend in clothing and the most recent viral cat video, but we aren't always aware of our bodies and how we take up space in the world. We are unaware of our surroundings, our environment, and our safety—until it threatens our well-being. We are unaware of how our actions impact others and, most disturbingly, are unaware that our daily movement habits impact the very people we are.

There are many things that contribute to our lack of awareness these days. There is a growing sense of entitlement and the need for instant gratification, both of which prevent us from being truly aware. When something doesn't go our way, or we feel that we are owed something, then we are unable to sit in the discomfort that comes with knowing we are not the center of the universe. When we feel uncomfortable we tend to distract ourselves or engage in unhealthy behaviors.

When was the last time you had a free moment and didn't pull out your smart device? As a society, we don't even give ourselves the opportunity to take in sensory information the way we used to because every free moment is filled with screen time. Our brains need down time and our bodies need our brains to sync. It may not operate on 5G, but the connection between your mind and body is *not* outdated.

**BODY AWARE BREAK** Take a moment to notice any distractions. What is preventing you from being truly present as you read this book? How many times have you checked your phone or even felt compelled to check your social media? Notice the distractions. Give them a place to exist in your mind and body. Simply paying attention to these distractions gives them permission to exist and then gives us permission to let them go.

Being aware is not like an on-and-off switch. To be *aware* means to have knowledge or perception of a situation. It requires a certain level of consciousness and the ability for reflection. And it doesn't only reside in your mind. It lives in your body: in the cells, tissues, organs, and muscles. So just because you choose not to think about something, doesn't mean it isn't impacting your life. In fact, these issues may be affecting your life more than you realize because your body is carrying them. "Your issues reside in your tissues," and unless you become aware of how they take up residence, they will continue to live inside you, impacting your every interaction as well as your physical and emotional health.

You make choices every day, often unconsciously, with regard to how you move your body. It is this ability to move or the suppression of movement that contributes to the awareness of your emotional well-being or lack thereof. You can take responsibility for much more of your mental health simply by bringing awareness to your body. Furthermore, you can improve your functioning and transform your life when you become *body aware*.

## Body Aware Defined

To be *body aware* means to have knowledge of your body and how it relates to your current situation or perspective. It is informed by *proprioception*, awareness of the position and movement of the body as well as the body's ability to sense itself in space; and *interoception*, the perception of sensations from inside the body. Being body aware entails being not just *mindful*, but *bodyful* to present sensations, feelings, and emotions that your body houses. The practice of mindfulness, which is what most people think of when learning to be more present, deals with using your mind to bring awareness to your body. Here, I am talking about using your body to bring more awareness to your mind, mood, and behavior.

Christine Caldwell, author, somatic practitioner and dance/movement therapist, coined the word *bodyfulness*.

> Bodyfulness begins when the embodied self is held in a conscious, contemplative environment, coupled with a nonjudgmental engagement with bodily processes, an acceptance and appreciation of one's bodily nature, and an ethical and aesthetic orientation toward taking right actions so that a lessening of suffering and an increase in human potential may emerge.[10]

To become body aware, one must have the ability to pay attention to signs and signals that the body gives off and then do something with that information. Being body aware means taking responsibility for one's existence and understanding that through the body, change is possible. Realizing that the body has knowledge, holds memories, and speaks using its own vocabulary is just the beginning to embracing a body aware existence. The body holds answers to questions the mind doesn't even know to ask. Learning the language of your body reveals these answers.

I would argue that being body aware is the single most important step to transforming your life. For anyone who has ever felt stuck in a job or a relationship; for anyone who feels they are living someone else's life or that they are destined for more, but feel trapped with no other options or alternatives, being body aware is the path to transformation—through *movement*. Let me say it again. How you move in your life has a huge impact on who you are and who you become. Your body has incredible knowledge and wisdom, but if you never listen to it—or even worse, spend your time silencing it—then you will never hear it. I am reminded of a client who at the end of our session turned to me and reflected that she spent so much time not using her voice that she forgot she had the ability to use it. You see, we become so accustomed to patterns of our communication—both verbal and nonverbal—that we forget we have options. We forget we have choices.

**BODY AWARE BREAK** What is your body trying to tell you right now? Notice any sensations? Is there tension between your eyes? Are your teeth clenched? These are all ways that your body is talking to you. Pay attention! It is there to help guide you to become a more enlightened, aware human being. It might be screaming at you, but if you start listening to it, that can easily become a gentle whisper.

## The Path to Becoming Body Aware

First, some disclaimers. While there are steps to becoming body aware, the most important piece is the process and the journey, as they are not a direct route but a winding, never-ending quest for self-awareness, unlimited potential, and a life of meaning and purpose. This path is not linear and often requires going backward or even sideways before going forward. I truly believe that a step back is *not* a setback.

Most important, everyone's journey is different and unique. While there are universal themes and common concerns, everyone's body is unique and therefore has its own movement preferences and affinities; much like a fingerprint, it is unique to each person. However, unlike a fingerprint, it can be modified.

Only you know what it is like to be in your body. *You* are the expert on you and this is only limited by your inability to be present to your needs, sensations, and movement patterns and behaviors. Everyone can benefit from embracing a body aware lifestyle, but several conditions must be present to lay the foundation for becoming body aware.

The first condition for being body aware is the knowledge that the trajectory of your life may be unsustainable. There must be recognition that the current state of affairs and how you operate are impacting your quality of life. This may be evidenced by abuse of alcohol, relying too much on unnecessary medications, exercising to the point of exhaustion, lethargy, a lack of agency, dissociation, or an inability to deal with life. When you can no longer manage the daily stressors of your life without relying on external validation, recreational substances, or overuse of drink and food, this is a clear sign that something needs to change.

The second condition for being body aware is the desire or willingness to change. It has been said that "your desire to change must be greater than your desire to stay the same." The desire and motivation to change must come from within the individual who wishes to reach their greatest potential. This is known as intrinsic motivation. While you may recognize the need to change, making those changes is not an easy decision or light commitment. This condition lays the foundation for taking responsibility and committing to your needs and health.

The third condition is recognition that there is a mind-body disconnect. The Buddhist tradition views the body and the mind as being dependent on one another. Latching onto Descartes's mind-body dualism, Western influence has perpetuated the separation of mind and body and now neatly packages the remedy. While mind and body have always been connected, we live in a modern society that has conditioned us to believe they are separate. This I believe is a main reason for the stigma that comes with mental illness, since it is often seen as less of a priority than physical health.

When we begin to understand that our mental health is shaped by our movement and that many physical ailments are manifestations of our mental health, then we might begin to treat them as equals or at the very least interconnected. Most people do not know that the potential for harmony exists between mind and body, and that by simply recognizing the inability to connect them, we can begin to embrace and reclaim a more bodyful approach to living and being in the world.

## Steps to Becoming Body Aware

So now that we know the conditions that must exist to embrace the practice of becoming body aware, let's examine the steps required to becoming body aware, all of which we'll explore in greater detail throughout this book. Four steps are required to embracing a body aware practice.

### 1) Recognize and identify current body vocabulary

We cannot know where we are going until we know where we've come from, so it is imperative that we identify current movement habits, patterns, and behaviors in order to know what is working and what needs to be worked *on*. Our body's vocabulary is the set of gestures, postures, expressions, really *all* movements that make up our movement profile— all of the ways in which we move including the qualities of those movements. Much like our personality traits and characteristics, our body movement has its own characteristics as well. Have you ever gestured a certain way and thought, "I'm turning into my mother!" Or recognized someone from a distance just based on their mannerisms and posture? While this will be covered in more depth in part 2, here are some ways to tune into your body's own language:

- Take time to notice daily movement habits.
- Keep a movement journal to track patterns.
- Check in with your body's sensations throughout the day.

## 2) Challenge your movement

We associate certain movements with certain people and they do the same for us. We rarely challenge these because they are familiar and comfortable, even though they may perpetuate unhealthy habits and behaviors. For example, when I limit my upper-body movement, this creates shallow breath, which often perpetuates anxiety. I may choose to engage in this movement because it allows me to take up little space and be less visible in a crowd. Perhaps visibility makes me anxious and I prefer to go unnoticed or undetected. We must identify our current movement vocabulary in order to recognize what movements are contributing to our current situation. Only then can we move onto the next step. Here are some suggestions:

- Become curious about the way you move.
- Try moving in different ways to challenge your current movement habits.
- Practice using your nondominant hand to drink, scribble, brush hair, etc.
- Cross your arms, legs, and hands, making sure to alternate between left and right sides.
- Play with different qualities of your movement like speed, tempo, and size.

## 3) Expand your movement repertoire

It is important that once we challenge the way we move, we practice these new ways of moving so that we learn to sit in and be okay with discomfort. This is where we build a healthy tolerance for emotional stress, increase our resilience, and enhance our ability to manage daily stressors. This is about actively engaging in new patterns, habits, and behaviors. This may look like:

- Walking a new path,
- Driving a different route,
- Standing/sitting in different postures or positions,

- Embracing hand gestures and other forms of nonverbal expression, or
- Trying a different form of exercise.

## 4) Integrate these movements into your daily life

Practice makes habit! The more you can practice different ways of moving, the more natural it will be to make them a part of your lived experience. Make a conscious effort to use these new movement patterns. Notice how it assists in your day-to-day operation, relationships, and communication.

## Body Aware in Motion

Erin, a young woman in her late twenties working in public relations, came to dance/movement therapy because she was in a perpetual state of anxiety. Erin reported feeling nervous and unsettled most days. She was always overanalyzing everything and never felt like she could relax. She had even convinced herself that her anxiety kept her safe from anything bad happening; so as long as she worried about something, everything would be okay.

Erin was eager to find ways to relieve her anxiety, but had tried years of Cognitive Behavior Therapy (CBT) and traditional forms of talk therapy with little success. She was skeptical about using movement and her body because of the fear and anxiety that it housed. How could being in her body actually alleviate the anxiety?

I invited Erin to map her anxiety. We started with a body scan, a somatic practice that guides an individual to check in with physical sensations from head to toe. Erin was able to go through her body and notice where she felt her anxiety and worry, namely in her chest and abdomen. She recognized these body parts and the intensity and quality of the feelings in each one.

As we continued, I invited Erin to notice if there were any places in the body that didn't house anxiety or worry. This puzzled Erin at first. She assumed that her entire body felt anxious. Taking her time to challenge this idea, Erin began to notice places where she didn't feel the presence of anxiety, such as her feet. I invited her to plant the soles of her feet on the floor in order to feel the support from the ground underneath her. Erin said that perhaps if those places always existed inside her, then anxiety wasn't necessary to feel okay. She could tap into the places inside where she felt the *absence* of anxiety and the presence of many other feelings. Together, we began to uncover those feelings that were masked by the anxiety, which was simply a security blanket.

## MOVEMENT RX: HEAD, SHOULDERS, KNEES, AND TOES

*Directions:* Find a comfortable place with limited distractions where you are able to focus on your body and your mind. This can be done by closing your eyes or simply focusing your gaze on a fixed point in front of you.

Bring to mind the age-old "head, shoulders, knees, and toes." Start by using those body parts as guides for bringing awareness to sensations in your body. Be sure to identify as many parts as you can that connect each region—for example, the neck, which connects the head to the shoulders. Be as detailed as possible in terms of checking in with your body. Your head includes your scalp, ears, eyes, nose, mouth, tongue, jaw, etc. Allow your body to move in any way it needs as you increase your awareness.

It is important not to assign "good" or "bad" to sensations but simply to notice them. If you hear or feel any judgments come up, just listen. This alerts you to how you assign meaning to sensations in your body. Notice the judgments or assumptions, and feel free to write them down.

*Dosage:* Weekly, biweekly, daily, or as needed.

*Side Effects:* Enhanced body awareness.

# TAKEAWAYS

* How you move impacts who you are and how you feel.

* We are unaware of how our actions impact others, and most disturbingly, that our daily movement habits impact the very people we are.

* "Your issues reside in your tissues," and unless you become aware of how they take up residence, they will continue to live inside you, impacting your every interaction as well as your physical and emotional health.

* The body holds answers to questions the mind doesn't even know to ask.

* How you move in your life has a huge impact on who you are and who you become.

# 2

# REDEFINING MOVEMENT

*To move is to live. To live is to move.*
—TONI SORENSON, author of *Redemption Road*

## How Are You Moving Today?

Yes, you read that correctly. I did not ask, "*Are* you moving?" or "*What* are you moving?" I asked *how.* Think how often you get asked, "*How* are you today?" The usual answers are *okay, fine, good.* But you rarely, if ever, get asked, "How are you *moving* today?" The fact of the matter is that we are always moving, otherwise we would not be living. In fact, the very absence of movement defines death.[1] At this very moment, your heart is beating, your lungs are expanding and contracting, your eyes are blinking, and thoughts are moving through your mind. There is even movement on a cellular level occurring all of the time, regardless of our awareness around this event. Food for thought: consider that how well you are living could be a product of how much you are moving.

The ways in which you are *not* moving say more about your functioning than the ways in which you *are* moving, and contribute greatly to negative mood, poor mental health, and untapped potential; all topics that will be addressed later on in this book. So I ask again: How are you moving? Still unsure how to answer that question? Keep reading.

> **BODY AWARE BREAK** Notice for a moment what parts of you are not moving. Has a body part fallen asleep? Have you been sitting in the same position for too long? Allow yourself a chance to move to a new position. Take a breath. Stretch out.

## Defining Movement

In order to redefine movement, it is imperative to look at conventional ways movement has been defined and the constraints in which we have been operating. Traditionally, movement has been defined as one, the act of physically changing the position of the body or its parts, and two, physically relocating the body. Let that sink in for a moment. It is not defined as physical activity or exercise or even a specific intervention. While its overarching umbrella includes exercise and physical activity, *movement* is so much more. All exercise is movement, but not all movement is exercise. We have become so conditioned to viewing movement as exercise or strenuous activity that we have forgotten all the ways our bodies move every day.

Katy Bowman, biomechanist and author of *Movement Matters: Essays on Movement Science, Movement Ecology and the Nature of Movement*, suggests that "we have outsourced so much movement in our society that we are actually losing evolutionary functions that were once necessary for survival."[2] *Outsourcing* refers to relying on machines or other people to do our movement for us. Examples of outsourcing movement would be buying chopped vegetables instead of chopping them ourselves, calling a neighbor on the phone rather than walking over to their house, or having our groceries delivered. In addition, we have outsourced so much movement that we overwhelm ourselves by trying to squeeze it intentionally into our day by going to the gym or taking a yoga class. Reframing our relationship to movement can put the ball back in our court and help us live with more purpose and meaning.

Movement is not just something you voluntarily, actively, or knowingly participate in. It is not just reserved for the yoga class you take every morning or the hour you spend on the treadmill at the gym. Movement is a part of every second of every day. It occurs whether you are aware of it or not, whether you welcome it with open arms or stubbornly resist it with every inch of your being.

Movement affects your physical health as well as your emotional, social, cognitive, and spiritual well-being. Your movement or lack thereof influences your relationships, your personality, your interests, and your life. Furthermore, movement is not just how or where you travel in space or even how much you exert yourself. It is how you sit, stand, gesture, sigh, breathe, exist. It is time to stop focusing on just *why* you move and also start looking at *how* you move. Once you identify how you move, you can begin to understand how the way you move influences who you are. Much like your parents told you that "you are what you eat," I encourage you to consider that "you are how you move."

Over the years, I have made it a point to ask people attending my workshops, "How do you move?" After the blank stares and looks of puzzlement wear off, the primary response is some type of exercise, for instance, running, jogging, dancing, yoga, etc. It seems to me that in Western society, we are so disconnected from our bodies that movement seems to focus around the external. We are unaware of the fact that movement comes from within and is not always about guidance or direction from a trainer, coach, or instructor. It can be about trusting our gut and moving from the parts of us that we didn't even know existed. We can begin to examine how movement is used for emotional and physical survival and how movement is our most primitive form of expression. And when we suppress or deny certain ways of moving, we actually deny ourselves from feeling our full range of emotions. When we deny our expression, we perpetuate suppression.

## Movement Is in the Eye of the Beholder

Perhaps we think of movement in terms of capability. If we are able to engage in large motor movements or regular physical activity, that is what we are primed to recognize. In fact, I know many people who will only move in certain ways because it feels good or will only do certain exercises because it is what they have always done. You may identify yourself as a runner, but does that mean that if you cannot run, then you do not exercise? What happens when your body movement is compromised due to physical or mental limitations? Should we dwell on what we cannot do and deny all the ways in which we are capable of moving, just to match our preconceived expectations—thus sacrificing our emotional and physical health?

Think about your association with movement and aging. Why is it that we accept that our ability to move deteriorates as we age? Just because the way we move changes as our body ages does not mean that we should stop finding ways to move every day. If anything, we should make more of an effort to keep moving in order to keep our minds sharp and our emotions regulated. Why is the culture of so many nursing homes around the country to allow older adults to sit lifelessly in front of TV screens, when we could be creating meaningful opportunities to engage using movement? Is it only when we are faced with a change in our mobility that we begin to recognize the micro-movements that we take for granted? Perhaps it takes the *absence* of movement for us to become aware of all the movement of which we are capable.

## How *You* Define *Movement*

Let's begin to look at how you define *movement* and how it plays a role in your life. Do you sit at a desk all day only to hit the gym in the evening? Do you go dancing with friends in the club on a Saturday night? Perhaps you take a morning walk or practice Tai Chi. These are examples of that physical activity I was talking about. But outside of exercise, would you consider yourself a "mover"? What does that mean outside of exercise?

How does it translate to your career, your social life, or how you interact with your environment? We often hear someone referred to as a "mover and a shaker." In the metaphorical sense, it is used to identify someone who gets things done, takes initiative, or even has influence over a field or activity. To best define movement, let's start in the body.

Think about all the ways your body changes position on a daily basis. The expansion of your lungs, the blink of an eye, every swallow; these are all ways in which your body changes position multiple times per minute. Every single thing your body does requires movement: digestion, immunity, reproduction—all of these functions require movement. As Katy Bowman said in her book, *Move Your DNA: Restore Your Health through Natural Movement,* "You can eat the perfect diet, sleep eight hours a night, and only use baking soda and vinegar to clean your house, but without the loads created by natural movement, all of these worthy efforts are thwarted on a cellular level, and your optimal wellness level remains elusive."[3] The World Health Organization defines optimum wellness as "a state of complete physical, mental and social well-being and not merely the absence of disease or infirmity."[4] In order to reach your optimum wellness level, it is imperative that you explore your current relationship to movement.

Movement can include rhythm, pace, direction, intention, tempo, shape, and size. Movement is not only innate to all animals, but it is our most primitive form of communication, a way to express ourselves, and a way to connect to the world around us. Our eyes are blinking, our hearts are beating, and blood is flowing through our veins. Truthfully, we have been moving since the moment we were conceived, as cells dividing. Once birthed, we are breathing and our hearts are beating to their own unique rhythms. It is this breath and heartbeat that become the foundation for exploring and connecting the mind and body. Through the mind-body connection, we have the power and ability to tap into and even enhance our experiences. Movement is not just about physical health or brain health. It is mental health. This is an opportunity to learn how to preserve it, protect it, maintain it, manage it, and most important, take responsibility for it.

## Influences on Movement

Consider the environments you come across on a regular basis. The office, your school, your home, even your community all represent different environments that your body interacts with regularly. Perhaps you have a long daily commute, sit in traffic as you drop your children off at school, or sit for eight or more hours in front of a computer screen. As I write this in 2021, I find myself a product of an environment I didn't necessarily choose. I along with the rest of the world am in the middle of a global pandemic that has completely changed the landscape of my social, emotional, and physical environment. The constriction I often feel in my body is a reflection of the restrictions I have placed on my social interactions. My days spent on Zoom or telehealth sessions have convinced my body to stay within visible range of a thirteen-inch screen. While I am not alone in this, it has been the ultimate test for me to embrace a body aware practice and to reflect on how I can intentionally move my body to alter my environment.

There are many external factors that impact movement. Our environment has the ability to restrict, challenge, and limit the way we move. The temperature in a room can cause you to curl into a ball to conserve body heat or to spread out in order to decrease your core temperature. Being in uncomfortable or compromising positions affects how you move, especially in relation to others. Consider how your movement is affected when you are in an environment that makes you nervous, anxious, or overwhelmed. Public speaking in front of a large audience is one example, and for many, this difficult and anxiety-provoking experience can lead to shaking, freezing, digestive reactions, or even fainting. Living in a stressful home environment, a cramped apartment, and during an ever-changing social and political climate all impact your movement. For some people, even being in an environment with too much space can be overwhelming.

Another factor that impacts movement is emotional health. We move differently depending on how we feel. When we are happy, our bodies are typically more relaxed, leading to slower or more indulgent movements.

If we are sad, our movements might become heavier, more restricted, and slower. Just like our emotions, our movements can have varying degrees of intensity and strength. These are examples of different qualities of movement that contribute to an individual's movement profile.[5] For purposes of this book, a movement profile is the set of traits, characteristics, gestures, and mannerisms portrayed by the body. Each person has their own profile that acts as a signature, a distinct form of embodied identification, if you will. This profile is made up of not just the movements themselves, but the nuances of the movements.

Lastly, consider how clothing plays a role on your movement. Tight jeans that constrict our ability to sit or bend our knees, high-heeled shoes that restrict the movement of our feet, and waist trainers or corsets that impede our ability to breathe are just a few examples. I am definitely from the camp that fashion is a form of expression, but my point is that we don't always take into account how what we wear impacts our movement and therefore perpetuates our current mental state or influences our overall mental health.

## The Qualities of Your Movement

Let's examine the qualities of your movement that make up your own personal movement profile. I do not just mean how well you are moving. In this context I am referring to characteristics or attributes of your movement. You have developed habits or patterns that have become ingrained in your body and hardwired in your brain. So what characteristics do you notice in your movement?

> **BODY AWARE BREAK** Focus on a part of your body that is actively engaged in movement. How is that part moving? What are the qualities or characteristics of that movement? Is that part of your body difficult to move? Does it feel heavy? Maybe it is relaxed and moves at a gentle pace. Can you identify a rhythm in that part? What is the tempo? Quick? Steady? Slow? Notice how you qualify the movement of that body part.

There are several models for noticing, qualifying, and even coding movement qualities that vary greatly depending on elements of culture, race, religion, and ethnicity. One such example is Laban Movement Analysis (LMA). Laban Movement Analysis is a "method and language for describing, visualizing, interpreting and documenting all varieties of human movement."[6] Laban was certainly not the first to observe movement and I want to make it clear that LMA is not the only way to observe and assess movement.

During my education as a dance/movement therapist, LMA was a focal point and required study for my program training. More recently LMA has endured criticism, not only due to Rudolf Laban's allegiances during World War II, but also for its Eurocentric focus that perpetuates oppression and minimizes the embodied BIPOC experience. Other movement assessment tools I am familiar with are Bonnie Bainbridge Cohen's Body-Mind Centering, Judith Kestenberg's Movement Profile, and Irmgard Bartenieff's Fundamentals. I recognize there are others, including necessary models that embrace the African Diaspora and African aesthetic, which I am still learning about and have not included in this book because they are out of my scope of knowledge and experience. Some resources have been included at the end of this book.

Keep in mind that movement observation and assessment are not about assigning meaning or judgment to a person's movements. They are a way to support the individual's understanding and exploration about how they move. I cannot qualify a person's movement without having a cultural frame of reference. While I see universal themes in movement qualities, the emotional contexts and interpretations are experience- and culture-specific. In chapter 5, I will explore more how universal themes in qualities of movement can facilitate emotional expression and support self-awareness.

While I am a product of my education, which I am currently dedicated to deconstructing with regard to oppression and systemic privilege, I associate qualities of movement with LMA. While studying LMA, I was first exposed to the idea of movement affinities—common or expected traits of movement. This, to me, essentially means that we continue to move in the same way due to habit or external expectations. This habit becomes so ingrained that we may be blind to how we are moving and unaware of how it impedes our daily functioning.[7]

Through his research, Laban found that embracing different movement patterns impacted productivity.[8] His research suggests that we can move our bodies to change our minds and we can change our movement habits to change the way we cope with and manage the world. Don't want to be so rigid in your decision making? Learning to embrace more fluid indirect movements may allow for that shift to occur. Finding it hard to focus and direct your attention? Consider inviting more direct movement into your body to support this need. This takes awareness, intention, and practice, but it is possible.

Movement can also be thought of in terms of how you approach life circumstances and situations. How you move through your life is yet another relationship to movement that we all have. This may feel out of your control, but I guarantee that you have more input than you realize. Your relationship to time and space influences how you move in your life. What is your relationship to time? Do you procrastinate or do you blow deadlines out of the water? How about space? Do you take up as much space as possible or do you keep to yourself and avoid touch altogether? This again will be explored further in chapter 5.

I am reminded of one of my first clients. Her own movement habits were preventing her from connecting to the world, others, even herself. What I remember most was not the words she spoke, but rather her stooped posture, poor eye contact, and hollow chest. As I sat across from her, the anxiety, discomfort, and lack of presence in her body was palpable; it was as if it were another person in the room. I could feel the weight on her shoulders as if it were mine, the emptiness in her torso, the absence of self-confidence in her eyes, and the anxiety in her limbs.

In addition to gathering information through typical verbal communication, I invited her to participate in a movement assessment. This could allow for both of us to observe her movement qualities or affinities, which could then illuminate her emotional resilience and mind-body awareness (or lack thereof). As a dance/movement therapist, this is what I have been trained to do: use the body to uncover psychological paradigms, preventing the person from living life to their fullest potential. The information we uncovered together shed light on where the work needed to begin.

I asked her to embrace her upper body in a hug. As she wrapped her arms around her upper body, she gently lowered her chin, covering her eyes and face with her elbows. I asked her how this felt and she said, "Safe, inviting, and protected." As I invited her to slowly open her arms, she managed to reach them to about shoulder width apart, palms facing toward each other, barely able to lift her chin and struggling to meet my eyes. When asked how this felt, she muttered, "Vulnerable," such a simple movement directive and yet so difficult to perform. Had I asked her to reach across the table and grab me a tissue or stretch her arms out in attempt to touch each wall in the room, she could have. She had no physical limitation that prevented her from opening her arms in any way. She did, however, have an emotional safety mechanism that kept her guard up. When I asked her to speak more to that vulnerable part, she expressed that she felt alone and truly believed that no one could ever relate to her experiences so she intentionally kept to herself and protected her heart for fear of getting hurt. Her body was protecting her and it had not only impacted her ability to connect but also it had actually changed the way she moved.

Why is this important? While traditional psychotherapy does not prioritize the body, it is a crucial piece to my process. Meeting a client where they are means meeting them in their body and observing how their movements or lack thereof play a role in their functioning. If most of our communication is nonverbal, then it is imperative that I pay attention to and acknowledge all the ways the body is talking.

You see, how you move further solidifies your core beliefs and vice versa. Dr. Nicole LePera, The Holistic Psychologist, defines a core belief as "a belief that is created in the subconscious mind between birth and age seven that a person has internalized as 'truth' or 'reality.'"[9] These realities become embodied and must be addressed in order to fully deconstruct whatever paradigms we see as "truth." In the instance of my client, she needed to acknowledge where her mind and body were with regard to her "truths" and then invite in the possibility of what different movements meant and how they challenged her reality.

Just like this client, I have seen individuals of all ages and abilities challenge this idea of *movement* as something more than physical activity. They embrace nonverbal communication and body language as a new way to uncover, express, and develop their beliefs, identities, and relationships to self, to others, and to their environment. So often we feel controlled or even manipulated by our own thoughts, which for some can be confusing, overwhelming, challenging, or even disturbing. We can reach our minds through our body's movement. How we move can allow us to change our thoughts, behaviors, and responses to various people, places, and situations. Just as our thoughts do not define us, neither does our movement. We can learn to adapt our habitual movements and in turn change our minds in the process. If our movements influence how our minds develop, then I urge you to consider how moving your body influences your emotional state. By moving your body, you can move your anxiety, depression, trauma, and other emotions. By moving your body in different, unconventional ways, you change how you take in and process information and how you cope with and manage emotions and the world around you.

We live in a world where mindfulness and meditation have become mainstream vocabulary, yet the practice still comes with the expectation of setting aside time or needing to implement a certain routine. Mindfulness starts within ourselves. Becoming more aware of our own bodies and how we move through our lives or remain stuck in them is where the work begins.

In a world where violence is more commonplace, at a time when we need to empathize with our neighbors more than ever, now is the time to explore our relationship to movement—to understand that it is more than physical activity and exercise. It is not just external. It is in everything we do. It is in our relationships, our jobs, our being. And, it is not just the movement we *do,* but more often than not, it is the *lack* of movement that holds the key to uncovering our greatest potential as individuals, communities, and as a society.

In order to redefine movement, it is imperative to acknowledge how disconnected we are from our bodies. In Western medicine, traditionally, mind and body have been treated separately. There is a global pandemic that seems to worsen as we engage and indulge in technology and other practices of convenience. Consider how we use *movement* in our daily language. It often seems to have a direct link to motivation, productivity, or lack thereof. We may hear "move on," "move over," "move out," even "move it." In the age of technology, emojis, and text messaging, we may overlook the many phrases in the English language that seem to suggest there is a relationship between movement and mental health. Consider these examples: "seeing eye to eye," "thinking on your feet," "bending over backwards," "getting something off your chest," or "a pain in the neck."

Many of these sayings and more used to be part of our everyday language, but even our verbal communication has become disembodied. We continue to perpetuate this mind-body disconnect, yet there are reminders everywhere that we need to listen to our bodies more than ever!

## Redefining Movement in Motion

I entered a memory care unit of a nursing home, and before I was able to introduce myself to the residents, the staff quickly made me aware of the residents who were chair-bound and "not able to move," let alone dance. This was not the first time I had encountered this, so I proceeded to introduce myself to each participant in the circle, making eye contact and reaching my hand out to say hello. Recognizing that the milieu housed pretty advanced cases of Alzheimer's disease, I knew it would be best to take it slow and allow natural movements to emerge from the residents as opposed to me directing them. Once I settled into my seat, I began to play some gentle music and immediately noticed many of these individuals tapping their toes. Participants who were sleeping when I first arrived had woken up and were wiggling their fingers, tapping their toes, beginning to make eye contact, and noticing me.

When the moment seemed right, I turned down the music and reintroduced myself to the group. I then took a moment to ask the group, "How are we moving today?" There was a brief moment of silence, and then one gentleman spoke up and said, "I am breathing." People nodded in agreement and smiled with approval. Another gentleman said "sneezing," while another participant said "coughing," and another said "hugging, kissing, chewing." Others chimed in, and before I knew it, everyone had shared one way in which they moved. I made eye contact with a staff member, whose eyes widened in disbelief. I smiled, turned the music back up, and continued.

## MOVEMENT RX: IDENTIFYING YOUR MOVEMENT

*Directions:* Write down all the ways in which you are moving right now. Think about the smallest movements that may be happening as you read this. Remember that we breathe on average 20,000 times a day. You can also start by identifying the places in your body that are still or feel disengaged. Then you can start to see the micro-movements that are occurring simultaneously.

*Dosage:* Practice for five minutes, three days a week, and work up to a daily practice.

*Side Effects:* Greater awareness of movement, mobility, and resilience.

# TAKEAWAYS

* How well you are living could be a product of how much you are moving.

* Movement is a part of every second of every day.

* Movement occurs whether you are aware of it or not, whether you welcome it with open arms or stubbornly resist it with every inch of your being.

* When you deny your expression, you perpetuate suppression.

* By moving your body in different unconventional ways, you change how you take in and process information and how you cope with and manage emotions and the world around you.

# 3

# YOUR BODY TALKS

*When the eyes say one thing, and the tongue another,*
*a practiced man relies on the language of the first.*
—RALPH WALDO EMERSON

Let's be honest: you cannot ask Siri or Alexa, "How am I feeling today?" or "What does my body need?" Only we can answer those questions for ourselves. The problem is that the more we connect to technology, the less we connect to ourselves and to what we truly need. We have become experts at the art of distraction. Reminder: what we lack in awareness, we make up for in distraction. As long as we are distracted, we never find time to focus on the body, which is talking all the time. Let me paint you a picture. . . .

I was watching TV with my daughter, Samantha, who was three at the time. She looked at me and said, "Mommy, my tummy hurts." My thoughts immediately started to race. *Is she sick? Is she going to vomit? Should I call her school and tell them she won't be there?* I tend to overreact when the health of my child is involved. I could feel the tension rising in my torso. I stopped my thoughts from spiraling by pausing and taking a deep breath. Here is how the conversation played out:

Me: *"Why do you think your tummy hurts?"*

Daughter: "My tummy is sad."

Me: *"Why is your tummy sad?"*

Daughter: "My tummy is sad because it is hungry."

This conversation stopped me in my tracks. My first thought was, *Holy cow, my daughter is already listening to her body! Dance therapist in training!* My second thought was, *How intuitive!* Giving my daughter the opportunity to listen to her body empowered her to solve her own problem. She didn't even have to Google the symptoms. All she had to do was listen, pay attention, and listen: I got her a snack and moments later she said, "Thank you, Mommy. My tummy is very happy now!"

Bottom line: it is imperative that we relearn to connect with our bodies to harness our potential for wellness and to manage our mental health. That's correct, I said *relearn*. The interesting thing is that we were born with this instinct, and somewhere along the road to higher cognitive development, we lost sight of how valuable the body's knowledge and wisdom really are. Of course this is difficult while we are plugged into our devices, rushing to meet a deadline, or taking care of our family. More important, we must allow ourselves to feel and sit in uncomfortable emotions in order to identify them and move through them. My daughter wasn't comfortable with a hurting tummy, but being with it and listening to it allowed her to meet a very basic need.

**BODY AWARE BREAK** Let's practice listening. Put down any distractions that you may be interacting with. Take a moment to focus on one part of your body . . . any part you want. First, notice any sensations in that body part (tension, tingling, stiffness, pain, etc.). Second, find a way to tend to that part. How? Simply by moving. Move the tension, the stiffness . . . give yourself permission to communicate with your body. What do you notice?

You see, we rely on our inner monologue to guide us—that "voice in our head," so to speak, that often gets confused for intuition. But there is a reason that we talk about a "gut feeling." It is not the mind that guides us but the body that senses and exists in this world that takes in stimuli and responds to it every second of the day. Why do we ignore it? Numb it? Minimize it? Because we don't want to feel pain. Pain is often seen as punishment, not as a signal from the body telling us to wake up and pay attention. The more we ignore it, the louder it screams.

With our distractions at an all-time high, we are afraid to sit in silence. It is *in* this silence that the mind often becomes loudest. The louder the mind becomes, the more we look to distract it. Your body hears everything your mind says. The body has the power to listen and quiet the voices, but if we don't know how to use it, we continue to numb, minimize, and ignore it.

What's the first thing you do when you get a headache or feel pain? Most people pop a pill. Have you ever thought to ask, "Why do I have a headache?" Your head is trying to tell you something, and the first line of defense is to silence it with painkillers. I'm not suggesting that painkillers are bad or even unnecessary. I'm merely suggesting that rather than it being the immediate response, it can become a conscious decision once we have listened to what our body truly needs; otherwise, that headache will come back. If we do not eliminate or even identify the cause of our pain and discomfort, it will remain. You will never resolve emotional issues if you do not address the body that houses them.

## Nonverbal Communication Reigns Supreme

Did you know that most of our communication is nonverbal? In his book, *Silent Messages: Implicit Communication of Emotions and Attitudes,* Professor Albert Mehrabian introduces the 7-38-55 rule. He states that 7 percent of meaning is communicated through spoken word, 38 percent through tone of voice, and 55 percent through body language.[1] That suggests to me that talking about an issue only communicates a small portion of what we actually experience.

So if approximately 90 percent of our communication is nonverbal, why do we continue to rely on words and formal language to express our issues, concerns, and sometimes our innermost secrets and thoughts?

Why, when a child is diagnosed with a verbal delay or sensory difference, do we immediately go to speech and physical therapy? Why not go to the *source* and meet that child in their senses? Meet them in the body.

Spoken language doesn't always express what we are truly feeling. In fact, our words can deceive. We can condition ourselves to believe certain truths that are often contradictory to what our body needs and feels. We can convince ourselves, reason, and find logic with our words, but that doesn't mean it is congruent with our body's language. Legendary dancer/choreographer Martha Graham said, "The body never lies. It is the barometer telling the soul's weather to all who can read it."[2] So this begs the question, What can I do to fully express and bring awareness to all the parts of me that contribute to my current situation? You see, it is not always about talking out our emotions but more about embracing them, honoring them, and giving them space to exist so they can move.

Our body has a language of its own. It is vital to listen to our body in order to achieve our most optimal level of functioning. Learning to listen to the body leads to greater emotional resilience, increased energy, and the ability to achieve your wildest dreams while remaining grounded, centered, and true to your process. Just like a toddler seeking attention, when we don't listen to our bodies, they have a way of trying to get our attention. Take for example the nagging lower back pain that you may experience after a long day on your feet or sitting at your work desk all day. It is your body's way of saying, "I am here. Pay attention." If we don't move, the tension builds and often turns into more pain or even inflammation. Furthermore, when we are out of touch with the sensations in the body or minimize their impact, we may lack the ability to identify when something is functionally or structurally wrong. When our bodies don't feel heard—or even worse feel ignored—just like that toddler, they act out. The body can lash out, shut down, or even go into "people-pleasing" mode.

Gemma was referred to me because she had been experiencing psychosomatic symptoms, physical ailments stemming from psychological issues. Gemma had also been experiencing panic attacks, intense anxiety, and blackouts for several months. She had aches and pains in her lower body that could not be explained by any medical doctor.

Gemma made it clear that she was no stranger to talk therapy and that she had spent years processing and working through sexual abuse and emotional trauma. On our first meeting, it was clear that Gemma was completely disconnected from and unaware of the lower half of her body. I anticipated that she might be holding onto the trauma that she had thought she'd already processed.

With her permission and on her own time, I invited her to stretch her back, arching and curving while on her hands and knees supported by the floor. As I was able to pinpoint the exact place in her spine where the movement seemed to freeze, I asked Gemma to focus on that part. I asked her, "If this part could talk, what would it say?" She paused and then proceeded to say, "It's lonely and it needs attention." That's exactly what we gave it. We made sure to pay attention to the parts of her body that were screaming for attention. As we uncovered her emotional pain, her physical pain subsided.

Gemma's *dis-ease* had led to *disease*. *Dis-ease* refers to a "lack of ease or comfort," while *disease* typically refers to sickness or the body's inability to function properly. In an article entitled "From Dis-ease to Disease," Marlene Jennings writes, "When the body is constantly in a high-stress zone over a longer period of time, that excess amount of cortisol within the body can bring about numerous unwanted symptoms."[3] This leads me to believe that disease finds the place that holds emotions we do not face. Consider an individual who has never opened their heart to love. For fear of rejection or intimacy for a myriad of reasons, what happens to this person's heart? Or similarly, someone who holds grudges, never letting go of anger or hurt. The anger acts as a cancer that fills the places in the mind and body that hold those feelings. Is it possible that these individuals are more susceptible to disease? Heart attack? Stroke? Cancer?

We know there is always a nature versus nurture debate and that disease isn't completely dependent on genetics. There is an environmental piece that I believe entails our emotional environment, the stress we endure or place on our system due to psychological paradigms. Think about the Grinch who realizes the power of Christmas and miraculously grows a larger heart. Fictional character or not, it seems valid that how we think directly correlates to our physical well-being. Consider how our movements influence how we think, and you can conclude that by moving differently, we can change our bodies' susceptibility to disease and illness. I am not suggesting that all disease is a result of stress and unresolved emotional issues. I am merely pointing out that there is a connection between emotional unrest and physical distress. I believe the parts of our bodies that carry the emotional load of our experiences are more susceptible to physical ailments.

You are the expert on your own body and your own lived experience. No one else knows what it is like to be in your body. Each part has its own voice and way of communicating. It's not as simple as typing symptoms into WebMD and getting a diagnosis—which I don't recommend, by the way. I am talking about an embodied knowledge that you can learn and practice, just like learning another language. Learning to interpret your body's communication style, rhythm, stress response, and movement qualities empowers you to advocate for your needs, identify your physical and emotional limitations, and set healthy boundaries that promote balance and integration. Remember, the body holds answers to questions that the mind doesn't even know to ask. All *you* have to do is listen.

## Body Language versus Your Body's Language

In order to uncover how to listen to your body, it is important to differentiate between body language and your body's language. Body language is one type of nonverbal communication in which physical behaviors (posture, gestures, and facial expressions) are used to relay information. Certain facial expressions, seven to be exact, can be interpreted and have a universal element that can be seen across cultures, genders, and demographics. Let me illustrate this point using an excerpt from an article entitled "Is Body Language Universal?" written by Janet Barrow:

> In 2017, a group of researchers from Dartmouth College conducted a study to determine how universal emotion-specific facial expressions are. They traveled to a remote area in the highlands of Cambodia, where a pre-literate group known as the Kreung live in isolation. This was

important to the investigation, as researchers wanted to be certain that their subjects' ability to produce or recognize specific facial expressions would not be influenced by interactions with outside groups.

With the help of an interpreter, a well-known performer of Kreung dance and music was asked to act out five scenarios representing five different emotions: anger, disgust, fear, happiness, and sadness. Soundless video recordings were taken, and these were later shown to 28 Dartmouth students and employees. They were asked to identify the emotions from a list of possible options. The results showed an 85% success rate—much higher than would be expected by chance alone. This suggests that certain emotional expressions may in fact be universal.[4]

American psychologist Paul Ekman developed an index of seven emotions that he deemed universal. These emotions, happiness, sadness, surprise, fear, disgust, anger, and rest, were based on a study conducted using over 10,000 photographs of facial expressions. More than 90 percent of all participants recognized emotions including happiness, disgust, and contempt.[5] (Note: this is not the same as movement observation and assessment, and while there are many body language experts, the title is not synonymous with dance/movement therapy.)

I remember a group therapy session that I facilitated in an adult day center with ten participants living with mild to moderate memory loss. All participants were oriented and verbal. One woman in particular stood out because she didn't speak any English. The staff seemed to make a big deal about this, but I knew that working in the body would transcend this "limitation." Mirroring her facial expressions, gently reassuring her through appropriate touch, and matching her own movement and rhythm allowed me to communicate with her without uttering a single word. Not only was this woman one of the liveliest participants, but the change in her affect from the beginning of the group to the end was like night and day. She entered the group quiet and reserved, but left with open arms and a smile that could brighten the darkest night. As I said goodbye to the group, she came over to me, gave me a big hug and said, *"Te amo."*

So what makes body language different from *your* body's language? We are not looking at universal movements that convey communication, but rather the internal signs and signals that *your* body expresses about its internal state of affairs. The body *expresses* what the mind *represses*.

Identifying your body's language is about you understanding your body and mind's internal state of being. Understanding your body's language means not only being aware of how your body expresses its internal state, but also an awareness of what the body is expressing externally. It is about translating your internal felt-bodily sensations, the physical visceral responses in your body like a hunger pang or a tight muscle, and identifying what they mean to you. I have adopted the phrase "speak your body." Much like the phrase "speak your mind," it empowers us to speak out, be heard, and validate our own truths even when words are not accessible. Why should the mind have all the power? Give your body real estate and invest in it.

Think of learning your body's language as learning a foreign verbal language. The only way to truly become fluent is to immerse yourself in conversation. That is ultimately what we must learn. We must strive to become fluent in the language of our bodies by practicing and engaging it in dialogue on a regular basis.

## Mind-Body Connection versus Mind-Body Communication

The mind-body connection isn't novel. Whether or not you are aware of it, it exists in you. Here's the thing, though: just because you have it doesn't mean you know how to access it, and if you don't know how to access it, then you are missing all the ways your body can assist in managing your emotional load. It comes down to understanding the ways in which your mind and body communicate with one another.

You may be familiar with different ways of learning. For example, some people are auditory learners, while others may be visual learners. I am coming to understand that my mind and body learn in different ways. And learning to utilize the connection between them means recognizing that not only does each process information in a different way, but that I must translate the information for both to be in alignment.

If you are anything like me, you live in your head. Even as a body-centered psychotherapist, I have a strong attachment to my headspace. I have begun to adopt the metaphor of being bilingual to explain my own process in understanding and utilizing my mind-body connection. I have come to realize that my first language is mind and my second language is body. As I have adopted a body aware practice, I have learned to consciously translate the information from my mind to my body. In my body I connect to an inherent wisdom and knowledge that my mind cannot comprehend or access on its own. Ever since I can remember I have had the need to analyze my experiences, or perhaps overanalyze them. It is probably one of the reasons I was drawn to psychology and psychotherapy. It seemed my body moved because my mind told it to.

Not only was I unaware of how my body spoke, but in most cases my mind was speaking for it, telling it what to do, and even making it doubt itself. If you have ever thought, "I wish I could turn my brain off," then you will understand just how loud and noisy our thoughts can get. In order to turn down the volume in my mind, I had to tune into my body.

**BODY AWARE BREAK** We are going to explore moving from the mind versus moving from the body. Begin by thinking about how you want to move and then follow that directive. For example, "I am going to take a deep breath." (Take a deep breath.) Try this for one to two minutes.

Next, just allow your body to move in any way it wants without the mind dictating it first. Again, try this for one to two minutes.

What do you notice? Is one easier than the other? Does your mind seek control over your body? When your body moves on its own, how does that feel?

Keep in mind that some individuals live in the body and have difficulty accessing the mind. For these people it is about consciously bringing the mind into the body. Either way, this communication is not necessarily quick. It takes time not only to identify which language is your native tongue, but also to become fluent. Fluency comes with practice. The speed at which I translate information from my mind to my body, while not immediate, is so much faster now than ever before. In fact, there was a time when the translation didn't occur at all. My mind and body spoke two different languages and had no way to communicate effectively. I was always in my head. Dance was the way that I physically relieved the emotional energy, but I'm not sure the underlying issues were completely addressed until I began to understand that the body itself needed to be a part of the healing process.

Want to acquire this skill for yourself? Here are five steps toward making that happen.

**IDENTIFY WHICH IS YOUR FIRST LANGUAGE.** Your first language may be "mind" if you find yourself overanalyzing situations, focusing on reasoning or logic, and trying to problem-solve. You may feel out of touch with your body, which would suggest an overreliance on the mind. "Body" may be your first language if you have difficulty putting your feelings into words or if you feel more connected to an experience rather than a discussion. There is no right or wrong. The most important piece is identifying which language feels more accessible and familiar.

**GET CURIOUS ABOUT YOUR "FOREIGN" LANGUAGE.** Now that you have identified which language is less familiar or feels foreign, so to speak, this is the time to ask questions and learn the culture inherent to that language. Find ways to interact with it, highlight it, or simply recognize the propensity to avoid it. Notice any judgments that come up around this new "culture." How can you practice humility for your own mind and body?

**INTENTIONALLY ENGAGE WITH BOTH.** Make an active choice to use the mind and the body. This can happen separately. This may look like spending more time in the mind by reading, journaling, or participating in cognitive games like puzzles or board games. On the contrary, find ways to be in the body by walking, exercising, and engaging your senses.

**CONSCIOUSLY TRANSLATE THE INFORMATION.** This means interpreting the information in the mind and the body. Notice how the mind and body each make sense of the same information in their own unique ways. Notice how certain thoughts create visceral responses in your body and how sensations in your body lead to certain thoughts. One example may be that when I think of all the things I have to do today, I feel my body constrict and tighten. On the contrary, when I notice my body is tight and tense, I think, "I feel pressured to do so much!"

**PRACTICE REGULAR CONVERSATIONS.** This means literally creating dialogue between the mind and body. Bring both into awareness and allow them to interact. Just like any language, if you want to become fluent, it takes time and practice. It also means finding the appropriate time. This will be harder to do when you feel distracted or overwhelmed. It is best to practice when you can really focus and pay attention. This may be a few minutes every day or thirty minutes once a week. Go at your own pace and just be open to the experience.

## Learning to Listen to Your Body's Language

Whether "body" is your first language or not, listening is the only way to really hear what your body is saying. Executing this step is *not* easy, but it is vital on the path to becoming body aware. I'm going to offer three steps that will allow you practice listening to your body's language.

1.  **DRAW ATTENTION TO YOUR BODY.** Find time throughout the day to tune into what you are experiencing and sensing in your body. Also known as felt-bodily sensations, these could be tension in the shoulders, tingling in your hands, warmth in your chest, or a jittery sensation in your legs. Whatever you notice, it is all valid. Here is a rhyme to help you remember to do this.

**HEAD, SHOULDERS, KNEES, AND TOES. MY BODY KNOWS.**

Write this down or keep it in your phone. Set an alarm as a reminder. Get into the habit of regularly identifying and listening to your body's sensations.

2. **IDENTIFY YOUR BODY'S VOCABULARY.** This means recognizing how your body likes to move or how it prefers to engage or disengage in movement. What movements are currently at your disposal, and which ones do you shy away from? Do you like to remain hidden and invisible, or do you want to be seen, take up space, and spread out? This will be discussed in further detail in chapter 5. At this point it is best to begin asking yourself these questions and creating awareness around your own movement habits.

3. **PRACTICE MEETING YOUR BODY'S NEEDS IN THE MOMENT.** This is perhaps the hardest step because it requires presence and action. Additionally, for those of us who ignore our body's needs, this will feel counterintuitive. Notice what your body needs and try your best to meet that need. Examples include getting a drink of water when you notice your body is thirsty, taking a screen break when your eyes feel fatigued, or giving yourself permission to slow down when your body needs a rest. This can also be accomplished by recognizing how emotions show up in your body and expressing them through movement. For example, I may stomp my feet when I feel angry or frustrated or wiggle my fingers when I feel agitated or worried. Chapter 4 will go into more depth on how to recognize a specific emotion and ways to express it.

These steps illustrate my own work with my clients. A client's mental health is prioritized and expression of emotion is facilitated by learning to involve and engage the body. We must go beyond words to confront life circumstances, diagnoses, and emotional issues.

I am reminded of one client, Sara, a fifteen-year-old high school student who struggled on a daily basis with overwhelming anxiety, which caused digestive issues, dizziness, and panic attacks. Upon entering the therapy session, Sara mentioned that that day was a particularly difficult day and her anxiety was a nine out of ten. I invited Sara to identify where in her body she was feeling her anxiety. As she put her hand to her stomach, I invited her to identify the rhythm and intensity of the anxiety. Sara began to vigorously rub her stomach in small intense circles. I encouraged Sara to move the rhythm to different parts of her body while focusing on her breath. Sara's movement began to morph into a gentle massaging motion down her arms. Her shoulders relaxed as she let out a sigh of relief. When asked to reflect on this experience, Sara mentioned that it was like learning to speak her body's internal language; trying to talk to it rather than ignore it.

## Why It Is Important to Be in Touch with Our Body's Language

Consider the following scenarios:

- A thirtysomething struggling with anxiety who has been in talk therapy for over ten years and has reached a plateau
- A young child on the autism spectrum who has difficulty expressing themself through verbal communication
- A family member who "doesn't want to talk about it"
- An individual living with dementia who cannot rely on verbal communication to express emotional and behavioral challenges

For these and a host of other reasons, talking is not enough. We must harness the power of the body's ability to communicate when words alone do not suffice. Have you ever heard the phrases "There are no words," "I'm speechless," or "Cat got your tongue"? Just because someone doesn't have the words doesn't mean the emotion or feeling doesn't exist. In fact, it is proof that emotions live beyond words. They live in the body and deserve to be expressed, heard, and witnessed. Remember that most of our communication resides in the body. If we don't acknowledge the body, we are doing ourselves a huge disservice. We are denying ourselves greater connection, empathy, and compassion. And it really speaks to how our own pain and unresolved issues impact those around us. Understanding our body's language opens the door to empathy. When we feel more in our own bodies we can feel what it is like to be in others' bodies. Repeat after me, "When I am in my body, I have a greater capacity to be with others in theirs."

Whether you have experience acknowledging your body or not, change is difficult. Give yourself permission to make mistakes and to fall back into old habits. Eventually, what will change is your ability to recognize when those old habits are coming back into play. And here's the kicker. At some point, those old habits will become the thing that feels uncomfortable. Your body will become an ally, and if you don't listen to it, it will remind you, forgive you, and help you get back on track.

## Times Are Changing . . . or Perhaps We Are

More and more clinicians, researchers, authors, and physicians understand that the body plays a huge role in mental health. This only solidifies the fact that talk therapy is not the end-all be-all when it comes to psychotherapy. If we do not take into account the body that houses our emotions, then we will continue to repeat the same patterns and behaviors, spinning our wheels and wondering why we aren't getting "better."

I firmly believe that traditional talk therapy, as we have come to know it, will be obsolete in the near future. That may sound harsh, so let me explain. I am not suggesting that talk therapy isn't valid or even effective. As a licensed clinical professional counselor, I am a talk therapist and value that skill tremendously.

What I am suggesting is that we are returning to our origins. The very definition of *psyche* is "the human soul, mind, or spirit." Webster's dictionary states that

> the word *psychology* was formed by combining the Greek *psychē* (meaning "breath, principle of life, soul") with *-logia* (which comes from the Greek logos, meaning "speech, word, reason"). An early use appears in

Nicholas Culpeper's mid-17th century translation of Simeon Partliz's *A New Method of Physick,* in which it is stated that "Psychologie is the knowledge of the Soul."[6]

Today, the field of psychology is concerned with the science or study of the mind and behavior, whereas psychology in its earliest forms meant the integration of body, mind, and soul. Somewhere along the line, we decided to disregard the body and soul and just began relying on the mind and not the embodied mind, but the cognitive processes that seem to reside from the neck up. As I mentioned in my own experience, often the mind speaks for the body or silences it altogether. We have been conditioned to believe that intelligence, wisdom, and "smarts" come from our ability to problem-solve, think critically, and analyze information. What about the wisdom and knowledge that come from experience? Actually feeling our way into a problem and moving through it rather than focusing on the need to solve it. This is mirrored in how our academia relies more on learning in a classroom as we advance into the system, rather than creatively accessing the body to support integration of information.

We are doing ourselves and Western society a great disservice by not incorporating the body and soul into therapeutic work. Only when we acknowledge the body can we then release and repattern the behaviors that limit our potential for change and growth. When we learn to move our bodies, we can truly move our minds.

## Your Body Talks in Motion

Molly was a mom of two young girls, and was a wife and a full-time executive. When we started working together she was on a medical leave from her job due to the immense anxiety she was experiencing. She contemplated admitting herself into a residential program but opted for an intensive outpatient experience instead. The first time we met I remember feeling like a part of her was missing—as if I was only meeting a small portion of the whole person sitting in front of me. I noticed in myself the need to emerge or run free.

She reported being hardworking and responsible, but also feeling lost. Since becoming a mom she stopped doing things for herself and only focused on her family's well-being and needs. Molly felt she was not taking care of herself, denying her body the movement it craved, and felt stuck in her head—a prisoner to severe anxiety. She even mentioned the strain that it was putting on her marriage. She wanted to reconnect to herself, and she knew the only way back was through movement and dance in particular.

Molly identified herself as a dancer since she was young. She took classes throughout college and even taught dance part-time before settling down and having a family. In our first session, after getting a brief history, I invited Molly to move around the studio and explore any movement possible. I encouraged her to listen to her body—ask it what it needed and how it wanted to move. After a few minutes, it was like a light switched on.

Molly began stretching her limbs, expanding her upper body, breathing deeply into her abdomen, and moving progressively through her spine. Her movements, which had been small and stiff, began to take on a flowy appearance, and there was a lightness in her torso. This went on for ten minutes. Her movements began to slow down and she found her way back to a stationary position. She took off her glasses and began to sob. She wiped her eyes, looked up at me, and said, "I feel like I found myself again. I really miss me."

## MOVEMENT RX: IDENTIFYING YOUR BODY'S LANGUAGE

*Directions:* Take a moment to identify an emotion you are feeling right now. Tapping into your felt-bodily sensations, write down what you notice.

Now, we are going to listen and talk to the body. Focusing on the emotion you identified, find a way to express it through the body. Perhaps the emotion has a rhythm, a pace, an intensity, or a gesture. Use any and all parts of your body to express that.

This is a practice in embodying your emotion. It may help to ask yourself, "How do I *know* I feel that way? If I couldn't use words, how would I express this emotion or how would I convey to others that I felt this way?"

Notice how your relationship to this emotion changes— what happens when the emotion resides in your body and not just your head?

*Dosage:* As needed.

*Side Effects:* Increased mind-body connection as well as ability to recognize and manage emotions.

# TAKEAWAYS

* It is imperative that we relearn to connect with our bodies to harness our potential for wellness and to manage our mental health.

* What we lack in awareness we make up for in distraction.

* You will never resolve emotional issues if you don't address the body that houses them.

* Disease finds the place that holds emotions we do not face.

* Only when we acknowledge the body can we then release and repattern the behaviors that limit our potential for change and growth.

# Part 2

# MOVEMENT IS A CATALYST FOR CHANGE

# 4

# MOVE YOUR BODY,
# MOVE YOUR MIND

*By placing the body in unique states,
we create pathways for fresh mindsets.*

—BRETT STEENBARGER, PhD, Professor of Psychiatry and
Behavioral Sciences, SUNY Upstate Medical University

Welcome to chapter 4, the heart of this book. After reading part 1, it is my hope that your personal connection to movement and your own awareness of your movement is evolving. Part 1 was all about identifying how you move, recognizing your own attachments to movement, and beginning to challenge or redefine what movement can be with regard to your mental health. Part 2 will explore how you can use movement—*not just exercise*—to facilitate pathways to new cognitions and behaviors, to uncover a broader movement vocabulary, and to unlock your cognitive potential. Movement is a catalyst for change and moving your body is the basis for facilitating that change.

> **BODY AWARE BREAK** Let's just sit with the word *change*. Notice what visceral reaction you have to the word. How does it sit in your body? Do you have a response? The idea of change can cause the body to freeze or tense up. See if there is a way to invite in some movement as you experience this response. How does your body move in the presence of change?

## What Is the "Mind"?

You can "be out of your mind," "speak your mind," "change your mind," "give someone a piece of your mind," you can even "lose your mind," but what *is* the mind? I guess it all depends on who you ask. The mind has been defined and redefined so many times, and still it feels elusive. For the purpose of this book, the mind is defined as the facet of an individual that allows them "to be aware of the world and their experiences, to think, and to feel; the faculty of consciousness and thought."[1] The brain is not the same as the mind; it is the organ located inside the human skull. As the brain develops, the construct of the mind develops as well, since our ability to think and feel grows and expands as the brain grows and expands.

I want to invite you to take a moment and identify for yourself where you feel your mind. You may have to close your eyes, and when you do, notice where you connect to your mind. You may feel it inside your head, encompassing the space around your head, or perhaps in another part of your body, such as the chest or the gut. This will be your own embodied sense of where your mind exists. I find this helpful, since the discussions and research around the mind can force us to stay in our headspace. Recalibrating the sense of mind ideally allows you to reset your focus toward the body.

## Early Movement Shapes the Mind

I distinctly remember early in my graduate program reading about developmental movement patterns and how they can influence the developing mind. I've continued to use that knowledge in my work today, and I have often wondered why it isn't more in the mainstream. Every individual completes certain developmental tasks within the body in order to function and express themselves fully. Furthermore, when these developmental patterns in the body are not realized, alternate patterns may form that do not fully support the next stage of cerebral growth—which can lead to physical or psychological issues down the road.[2] I found this intriguing, to say the least, and it has become the foundation for much of my work.

Keep in mind that skipping a developmental body pattern is not the same as having a developmental difference. Developmental milestones refer to behaviors or physical skills present in children as they grow. For example, a developmental milestone is an infant rolling over. Generally speaking, a developmental body pattern that provides the foundation for this milestone involves the connection between the head and tail(bone) also known as Head-Tail Connectivity, which will be described in depth further into this chapter. Developmental body patterns are the movements that support these milestones.

Anyone, no matter their cognitive or physical ability, can have unrealized developmental patterns in the body. Unless you are trained in or have experience in movement observation and assessment, movement analysis, or movement profiling, these unrealized developmental patterns often go undetected. The key point is that these embodied patterns are shaped by our early experiences and movements and lay the groundwork for how we interact with and make sense of our world as adults.

From the moment of conception, movement is present. Birthed into the world, we make sense of our surroundings and communicate our needs without a single word. As we engage in our environment, it is through movement and felt-bodily sensations that allow the brain and therefore the mind to continue to develop. In her book, *Making Connections: Total Body Integration through Bartenieff Fundamentals,* Peggy Hackney writes, "The baby manifests itself by moving, always moving."[3] Through tactile stimulation, feedback from people, places, and things, as well as experience, the brain takes in information and grows, connects, moves. From the beginning of our physical existence, I hypothesize that first comes movement, then comes the mind. Maria Montessori, founder of the Montessori educational program, was quoted as saying, "Watching a child makes it obvious that the development of his mind comes through his movement." Additionally, movement conveys what we think and feel. Bonnie Bainbridge Cohen, founder of Body-Mind Centering, says, "The body is the instrument through which the mind is expressed."[4]

Let me give you some examples. Neurotypical, physically abled infants learn to sit up on their own by six months of age, give or take a few months. In many instances today, infants are placed in devices such as strollers or high chairs that allow them to sit up before that developmental pattern is accomplished, leading to alternative patterning in the body. The child is supported by an external apparatus rather than from its internal musculoskeletal system. This can lead to lack of core support, which can have ramifications physically as well as psychologically as the child matures. While long-term effects are still unknown, research has shown that positioning devices do impact infant leg movements.[5] Physically the child may experience low muscle tone, while psychologically this can interfere with expression as well as impact the child's ability to be open and to build trust.

Now consider a baby on the verge of walking. The psoas muscle (pronounced *so-as*) is responsible for commencing movements associated with walking. The psoas, the only muscle connecting the legs to the spinal column, is the core-stabilizing muscle located near the hip bones that has been known to affect stability, mobility, balance, and flexibility. Research indicates that in addition to structural health, the psoas is imperative to our psychological well-being.[6] Liz Koch, author of *The Psoas Book,* states that our psoas "literally embodies our deepest urge for survival, and more profoundly, our elemental desire to flourish." If not adequately developed early in life, this can impact our emotional state, interpersonal relationships, physical pain, and ability to manage stress later on.[7] This resonates deeply with me, as my one-year-old son is learning to walk. It has been interesting to see how his venture into walking has paralleled his emotional development to express his needs and manage big emotions. This is an early illustration of how our movement or lack thereof can support emotional development.

These examples are here for you to begin to challenge how your body influences your mind, how the way you move impacts the experiences and relationships you encounter. That being said, there are so many variables that come into play. Plenty of individuals will live meaningful connected lives regardless of their body's adapted developmental patterns. For people who are looking to change and have not explored how their body may be keeping them from making those changes, this viewpoint can make all the difference.

Irmgard Bartenieff, dance theorist and pioneer of Westernized dance/movement therapy, said that "the essence of movement is change."[8] Bartenieff developed her own set of principles and exercises called Bartenieff Fundamentals. Drawing from her studies with Bartenieff, Peggy Hackney integrated these practices with her study of the developmental movement patterns of Body-Mind Centering that she studied with founder Bonnie Bainbridge Cohen to create what she calls the "Fundamental Patterns of Total Body Connectivity." These six developmental movement patterns provide an early foundation that supports brain development and expressivity. With regard to Bartenieff's work, Hackney states, "Functional capacities underlie expressive capabilities."[9] Without mastery of these patterns, later development can be impeded, and expressivity may be limited—meaning our emotions and the ability to express them will be impacted. Hackney's patterns are as follows:

- Breath
- Core-distal connectivity
- Head-tail connectivity
- Upper-lower connectivity
- Body-half connectivity
- Cross-lateral connectivity[10]

The following is a very basic breakdown of these movement patterns, in an effort to make them digestible and relatable to your needs and lives. Please note that this is my personal interpretation. If you are interested in a more comprehensive look, be sure to see the resource section at the end of this book.

Breath, while involuntary and unconscious, is the groundwork for all consecutive patterns. Hackney says, "Healing of the Body-Mind is directly connected with restoring full functioning respiration."[11] When we are not breathing fully there are physical and psychological implications. Take a moment and hold your breath. Notice what happens in your body when you limit your ability to breathe. This may include tension in the chest, lightheadedness, or a sense of panic. Now consider the long-term effects of this. This can impair our sleep, contribute to stress, and lead to brain fog and other cognitive dysfunction. Our existence and survival centers around breath therefore, it is the foundation for all connection.

Core-Distal Connectivity is a pattern focused on symmetry with the locus of control coming from the middle of the body. This provides the foundation for what we know of as a supported core or what Hackney terms as "Core Support." Bainbridge Cohen states, "In the human, the navel functions as a primitive center of control."[12] Quite literally it is the first connection we have inside the womb. All sustenance comes into us through our navel. This pattern is about the coming into and away from the center, exploring mobility and centering even before birth. This pattern helps create a personal home base as well as a sense of purpose later in life.[13]

Head-Tail Connectivity is all about the spine. A spine that can effortlessly access the vertical while also managing to be fluid and flexible reinforces a sense of self and grounding as well as establishes connection to the Earth and the environment. Hackney says, "All movement, from simple to complex, is aided by awareness of relationship through the spine."[14] This is the connectivity or lack thereof that contributes to the Westernized mind-body disconnect. When we are unaware of our spine, we are out of touch with ourselves and lack self-awareness.[15]

Upper-Lower Connectivity explores the relationship between the upper regions of the body and the lower regions of the body. Differentiation of each half is needed in order to foster collaboration. Large tasks to be learned in this pattern are "learning to set boundaries, learning to give and receive, [and] learning how to support your reach for the goal with a push that will get you there."[16] Inadequate patterning can lead to "a constant sense of failure" or a feeling that your "actions are meaningless."[17]

Body-Half Connectivity is essentially about stability and mobility. It is quite literally one side or half of the body providing support while the other half can move freely.[18] Psychologically this pattern explores opposition and recognizing where an individual "stands on an issue."[19] It can also be about feeling stable enough to explore other views or perspectives while remaining true to one's own opinions.

Cross-Lateral Connectivity refers to creating passages "diagonally through our core, enabling us to cross movement in a connected way from one side to the other as well as up and down and forward and back."[20] Examples are climbing a ladder or everyday walking and marching. This is the most advanced body pattern, as it results from the realization and culmination of all other patterns. According to Hackney, once this connectivity is realized, the possibilities in "human movement potential"[21] are endless; more on this in chapter 6 where we will explore potential through movement.

This brief breakdown begins to explore how inadequate patterning can impact adulthood. For example, the inability to distinguish "self" from "other," which is developed through early connections to the center or navel, can result in poor emotional boundaries. Additionally, lack of core support created through insufficient breath and spinal mobility can result in too much or too little tension in the body, which correlates to the inability to take action or advocate for oneself. There are so many psychological implications resulting from inefficient or mispatterned bodies. This is why moving the body is vital when looking to change current behaviors and thoughts. Changing your thoughts alone is not enough because it doesn't rewire the inept developmental movement patterns that have led to your current way of thinking.

Cognition has reigned supreme in the psychology space for a long time. Interventions like Cognitive Behavior Therapy (CBT), the "gold standard" in psychotherapy, suggest that we can change our cognitions in order to change our behaviors, but what about the body? Is it safe to assume that when we change our thoughts, our bodies adjust in the process? Not necessarily. While an improved mood can positively influence our posture, it might not become our new way of being.

Emotional issues will never be resolved without addressing the body that houses them. How those issues exist, live, and take up space in your body must be acknowledged as those are literally rooted in your being. Roots often run deep, so it is going to take more than trying on a movement to see permanent change. This is one of the reasons I challenge "power posing."[22] Power posing is a self-improvement technique where people stand in a posture that they mentally associate with being powerful, in the hope of feeling and behaving more assertively.[23] While I definitely see value in engaging in postures to conjure up a feeling, especially when we are looking to enhance our confidence before public speaking or boost our self-esteem before a job interview, there is an underlying assumption that the body trying on the pose is wired to access those feelings. That is not always the case. I cannot ask someone to try on an emotion or feeling they have no access to. Remember that what we think in our minds is developmentally wired through the body and those patterns must be addressed to make permanent changes. It is why sometimes we feel like we are just "going through the motions." That's because we are!

So what are some reasons that a person would not have access to an emotion? Quite frankly, because it wasn't modeled or accepted as they were growing up. We know that the body's language is a vital component to becoming body aware, but in order to tap into that language we have to understand what causes us to deny, silence, and suppress that voice. While there are many reasons, most traumatic in nature, I believe it is necessary to briefly discuss how these events influence our movement and therefore directly impact our developmental movement patterns.

## The Impact of Traumatic Events on Movement

Let me preface this section with the fact that trauma is not the focus of this book. There are so many amazing books and resources about how trauma impacts the body. Many of these will be listed at the end of this book. However, they don't directly talk about how trauma influences the ways in which we move with regard to patterns of movement. Most often they focus on what physiologically occurs in the body and how movement can be used to manage and even overcome our traumatic histories. I think it is imperative to talk about how our movement habits and patterns change because of trauma.

Trauma literally changes our brains, but more important, influences how we move. Without that awareness we will remain physically stuck in patterns of fight, flight, and freeze. In her framework of Restorative Movement Psychotherapy (RMP), the creator of Polyvagal-informed somatic and dance/movement therapy, Dr. Amber Elizabeth Gray says, "Relational trauma can literally force us to take a shape that is not our own."[24] Gray's work supports that qualities of movement discussed in the next chapter, weight, space, and time, are all influenced by trauma—how much weight we bear, space we take up, and time needed to engage or disengage with what we choose. Modifications in our movement are the foundation for emotional and psychological changes. By accessing elements of weight, space, and time—which Gray calls "portals of embodiment"—individuals can restore "a sense of belonging and meaning" after life-altering events. This is one of the many reasons that non–body-centered therapies alone do not support the restorative process, because as Gray mentions, "the imprint of fear is in the body."[25]

This is a vital point because not only does trauma change the body's movement, but also it can alter our reactions when emotionally triggered. Hackney mentions that "in trauma the organism often reverts to more primitive patterns of accommodation and adjustment."[26] This means that when we are emotionally triggered, we can resort to younger patterns of thought, speech, and movement. We can witness a mature, self-sufficient adult act out like a rebellious teen or belligerent toddler.

I am reminded of a client who had been in and out of treatment for disordered eating. During a particularly difficult time, she thought about going into a residential treatment center. I remember discussing potential options when I realized that all of the facilities I had named were for individuals less than eighteen years of age. I had forgotten that this client was well into her forties because all of her mannerisms and body language suggested that of a much younger individual. She was so engulfed by her trauma from a young age that it was showing up in her body and impeding her movement patterns.

Congenital birth defects, brain injuries due to tragic accidents, war, natural disasters, physical and emotional abuse, and systemic racism and oppression are just a few examples of trauma that directly impact the body. The body makes accommodations and adjustments in order to stay safe or to preserve what feels like safety. And the notion of "moving" out of that comfort zone can be even more terrifying than the traumatic event itself.

Accessing movements, especially when they signal early movement patterns, can bring up memories and feelings, both joyful and traumatic in nature. Dr. Candace Pert says, "Repressed traumas caused by overwhelming emotions can be stored in a body part, therefore affecting our ability to feel that part or even move it."[27] Ironically enough it is through the body that we can learn to access these emotions and move ourselves toward safety. In what Gray terms *Ground in the Swirl,* which alludes to finding stability in unstable or uncertain times, she offers the following movement interventions designed to create safety in the body.

**START EVERY DAY WITH A RITUAL.** Gray suggests beginning each day with an activity or practice to anchor and ground the body and mind. This becomes a way to find stability and predictability, even when life or our nervous system offer anything but that. This can be a physical practice like stretching or even a morning cup of coffee. Consistency is the key.

**PRACTICE "REGULATION BREATH."** While there are many breath practices, this one in particular focuses on the sternum. Drawing attention to the "heart's shield" allows the individual to shift into helpful directions. When we are hyper-aroused, breath can help us find rest and calm. When hypo-aroused, it can support energy and movement. To engage in this practice, place a hand gently over the sternum while breathing and apply a little bit of pressure, inviting in the opportunity for awareness through micro-movements of the chest.

GIVE YOURSELF THE "OXYTOCIN HUG."   Wrap your arms around your torso and gently rock. This boost of oxytocin aids in regulating our emotional responses as well as supporting trust, empathy, and positive communication.[28]

These interventions allow an individual to regulate their nervous system, find balance, and create a sense of calm in order to "promote comfort and ease during dis-ease or discomfort." This moves the body toward safety as it learns to neurocept, or subconsciously detect harm, more accurately through the process of physical and psychological recalibration. When this safety is established and accessible, the ability to challenge the adapted movement patterns becomes possible.[29]

I feel it essential to say that with regard to trauma, working in the body, while necessary, must be done gently and with great intention. Of course, when processing trauma it's best to work with a knowledgeable facilitator to support a safe atmosphere physically and psychologically for the mover, since safety and trust are vital for repatterning and rewiring the nervous system.[30] It is through this repatterning and rewiring that we can find the ability to speak our truths and embrace an embodied existence.

## Speaking from Your Body

I believe the lack of awareness around how our early movement patterns influence our mind is a huge reason why so many people plateau in traditional talk therapy. It focuses solely on expressing the mind through speech and vocalization. Bainbridge Cohen, developer of Body-Mind Centering, says, "We vocalize what we hear, based on the neuromuscular patterns established in our breathing and movement."[31] For most people, speaking is an unconscious process. There is no need to become aware of it as long as it is in working order. Ironically, one of the most common client concerns I have come across in psychotherapy is voice, the inability to "speak the mind" or feeling minimized or silenced. It's one of the very reasons I have made it a point to ask clients, "What's on your body?"

Vocalizing the mind only takes us so far and that is assuming we have the ability to access that voice. It's quite possible that others have always spoken for us, told us that our voice didn't matter, or that a life circumstance took our ability to speak our needs. The ability to speak is more than just having a voice box. It is also about believing that what you have to say matters.

It is through the body that permanent change occurs, ultimately bringing new patterns of thought and speech. Identifying insufficient patterns related to breathing, sucking, and swallowing provides opportunity to repattern more efficient breathing, digestion, and even vocal tone.[32] By physically engaging the body through early developmental patterns and identifying qualities of your movement, you can go from "going through the motions" to embodying and expressing your emotions.

We must address how the body is wired, or in some cases "miswired," to fundamentally rewire the mind. A body that is stretched by new experiences changes the mind's dimensions forever. When we challenge our ingrained movement patterns, as underdeveloped or alternative as they may be, we can navigate and rewire the psychological patterns in our minds. We can free ourselves from the fear, anxiety, doubt, guilt—everything—that keeps us from living productive, meaningful, and connected lives.

## Moving on Up!

Psychotherapy has traditionally involved accessing areas of the brain responsible for "higher thinking," which also happen to be the structures that are more advanced from an evolutionary perspective. Dan Siegel, *New York Times* best-selling author and executive director of the Mindsight Institute, says, "The 'higher structures,' such as the neocortex, at the *top* of the brain, mediate 'more complex' information processing functions such as perception, thinking, and reasoning," while the lower more primitive regions of the brain, which include deep within the brainstem, regulate basic elements like breath and heartbeat.[33] These lower regions are the first to develop in the womb and are therefore considered the most primitive.

This relates to what psychologists refer to as top-down and bottom-up processing. Top-down processing is theory driven and occurs when our previous knowledge or expectations influence our perception. Bottom-up processing, which is data driven, occurs when a stimulus influences our perception, and it is that perception that directs our cognitive awareness.[34] Quite literally the information moves up from the stimuli to the brain where it is interpreted. An example of bottom-up processing would be stubbing your toe on a piece of furniture. This involves sensing pain, which is then processed by your brain. Top-down processing would be avoiding that piece of furniture so as not to endure that pain again. Again, one is theory and experience driven while the other is data or sensory input driven.[35] If there is no prior experience to draw from, or your ability to access previous experiences is compromised due to stress, overwhelm, or trauma, it would make sense to approach emotional processing from the bottom up, beginning with current input of sensory information. When I speak of bottom-up in this sense I am referring to accessing both the lower parts of the brain and the lower parts of the body—particularly the chest, gut, and legs. When we literally drop into the body we encourage feeling and sensing from the bottom up, cognitively and physically.

If reason and logic are inaccessible due to a dysregulated nervous system or feelings of high anxiety or stress, it makes sense to change the focus from the top parts of the brain to the lower parts in order to facilitate self-regulation. Movement taps into the lower structures of the brain, which existed way before logic and reason became the boss. Our ability to manage and cope with our emotions becomes possible not through analytical thought and reasoning but through sensing and feeling our way up toward the higher regions of the brain. Self-regulation and emotion management are associated with the limbic system, which is centrally located. It can be very difficult and near impossible to access those parts from the top down. This suggests that processing emotions must start in the lower regions of the brain, the ones accessible through movement, and *move* their way up in order to be able to reason and think our way out of a problem. Essentially we must *feel* our way through in order to *think* our way out.

## Facilitating Change through the Body

Let's look at a body aware approach to creating change through movement. Try this: Make a fist with one hand. Now allow that fist to shift into an open palm. Congratulations! You have just facilitated change. It may seem to some that I am oversimplifying the connection between experiencing a change in the body and creating lasting change in the mind, but we have to start somewhere. When a person is fearful or hesitant to embrace change, tapping into movement in its simplest forms—like shifting our posture, lifting the head, or stretching the arms—makes change accessible and less daunting. This is different from the phenomenon of power posing, which usually starts with the feeling or emotion you are trying to invoke. I am talking about physically shifting the body to create postural change. It doesn't require implementing a new workout routine or taking up daily meditation. As previously stated, it requires becoming aware of how your body is currently patterned and actively inviting in and identifying new ways of moving.

Joseph Pilates was quoted as saying, "Change happens through movement." Change is essentially a shift or modification. There is often fear accompanied with change because it challenges that status quo that so many of us cling to for security and safety. Movement is an extension of the Self, and therefore a change in movement impacts who we are. How we move connects to how we communicate, relate, and interact with ourselves and the world. Change your movement and those things change as well. This is perhaps the scariest part of change. Changing who we know ourselves to be, who others know us to be, and even more so, acknowledging that we want to be someone or something else—something more—can be scary. With change comes grief or loss of what was and anticipation of what will be. That is why I believe if we can get back to the body and how it moves, we can create opportunities to see change happening in real time and know we are fundamentally safe and supported.

For so many people, conscious intentional movement feels unnatural. They have spent so much of their existence on autopilot—frozen, numb, dissociated, or in denial. The idea of moving when under stress feels counterintuitive and downright uncomfortable. I personally have lost track of how many times a client has uttered the words, "I feel stuck," or some variation of that. Whether it is emotional paralysis, freezing up, or even a loss of motivation, these all speak to an inability to *move*. The mind and body are emotionally and often physically immobile. Newton's first law of motion says that "a body at rest tends to stay at rest" unless an outside force acts upon it. What if that outside force was your own intrinsic motivation? Your willingness and eagerness to change your current situation must be greater than your fear of the change itself. Be the change you want to see in yourself by changing the way you move.

I was working with a young man who had endured an injury to his arm a few years prior. He was realizing that while the arm had healed, the emotional scars had not and this was impacting his daily life. No stranger to chronic pain, he had been conditioned to ignore it. From a young age he was taught to mask his pain and "be a man." He never allowed himself to sit with it because it was too overwhelming and "unproductive."

After many sessions of mostly talking with little ability to engage in intentional movement, we began this session with a body check-in. He immediately noticed a burning sensation in his arm. Suddenly he tensed up and mentioned that he couldn't move. "I feel frozen," he uttered. This had happened before and his habit was to dissociate from the physical experience—minimize the discomfort and change the subject. This would result in him closing his eyes, wrapping his arms tight around his torso, and shrinking. He would retreat back and lower his head.

Today was different. While "frozen," he remained present to the experience. His eyes remained open and his spine remained lifted. I invited him to notice what was happening in his body. He went on to explain that he was afraid acknowledging the pain would make it worse. Our work together had opened his eyes to just how much the fear was controlling not just his thoughts, but his posture and physical expression. This was the first time since the injury that he was present to the pain. And to his surprise listening to it allowed it to shift. He suddenly realized that his body was moving again, moving through that "stuck" place. His arms relaxed, his torso softened, he took a breath, and let out a sigh of relief.

> **BODY AWARE BREAK** Take a moment and interlace your fingers, ultimately clasping your hands and touching the palms together. Notice which thumb is on top of the other. Starting with that thumb, switch so that the other thumb is on top and successively switch all other fingers. How does this feel? How long can you stay there and allow yourself to feel what I can only assume is weird, strange, and likely uncomfortable? Shake out your hands. Now cross your arms. Again notice which arm is on top of the other. Now switch so the current one on top becomes the one on the bottom. How does this feel?

Your body is accustomed to certain movements that have been hard-wired into your brain. You sit in ways that are comfortable and familiar and rarely, if ever, challenge them. Doodling with your nondominant hand or sitting with your legs apart rather than crossed are just two examples of how you can begin to prime your mind by changing the way you instinctually and habitually move. The first step is to acknowledge what it currently feels like to be in your body.

## Meeting Your Body Where It Is

Think back to part I, where you identified your body's language. This is the foundation for being able to support your own needs through movement. This is what allows you to meet your body where it is so you can authentically find your own way of connecting to the emotional constructs in your mind. Chances are that by the time your mind is thinking it your body has been feeling it for longer. So what does it mean to "meet your body where it is?" Dance/movement therapist Dr. Jennifer Frank Tantia says, "You cannot know what you need until you know how you feel,"[36] and we don't know how we feel until we check in with our sensations and meet our needs or lack thereof by examining how they manifest in the body.

Observing and assessing how you feel through the body is necessary to implement change. This creates a baseline or starting point from which you can assess your own growth. As a dance/movement therapist, I don't simply tell my clients how to move. I start by inviting in the possibility of movement and allow each person to embrace the movement that is possible for them in the moment. It's often about moving from the places inside you that you didn't even know were there. It becomes about meeting the body where it is in order to guide the mind where you want it to go. Accessing what you *want* to feel is only possible when you know *how* you currently feel. Supporting where you are in the current moment through the body is invaluable. It can also be the hardest because it often requires that we sit in discomfort.

Therapists often refer to "meeting a client where they are (at)," which means being present to the client's needs, not pushing an agenda, and not bringing the client into exploring or processing an experience that they are not willing, ready, or capable of exploring. While this is an invaluable skill and the mark of a great therapist, it is not proprietary. This skill of being present to current feelings and emotions is accessible to everyone. All too often we minimize, deny, or numb our own experiences. We need to redirect our focus from thinking our way out to feeling our way through. When you feel stuck emotionally you always have the option to move physically. However, when you are feeling frozen, stuck, or immobile, movement seems inaccessible and impossible. The only way through it is to go into it. Such was the case with a client I once had who commented on how unnatural it felt to move. She associated movement with visibility, which completely overwhelmed her. Her M.O. in life was to fly under the radar and go undetected. This entailed wearing baggy clothing, dark colors, covering her eyes with her hair, and keeping her body movement as limited and as small as possible.

In one particularly difficult session, during which she was struggling with her anxiety, she had literally made herself as small as possible sitting on the couch in my office, crying. The more she cried the smaller she became; her knees pulled up into her chest, her arms wrapped around her legs, and her face sunk into her knees. We began by acknowledging and noticing how small and tight her current posture was. I asked her to verbalize what she felt. "I feel tense and anxious," she whispered. I invited her to focus on a part of her body that felt the least tense. She began to wiggle her toes. These micro-movements of her feet brought awareness to her legs. This allowed her to notice just how tight her lower body was, which was perpetuating the lack of movement in her torso as they were compressed together in this upright fetal position. She loosened the grip she had around her knees. This slight shift allowed her to move into a less closed position, allowing her chest to expand and take up space. She began to visibly breathe and was able to lift her head and make eye contact with me.

Meeting her body in its tension and anxiety fostered her ability to be present. As unnatural as movement felt, she authentically moved in a way that validated her emotions, enabling her to shift her perspective.

So what if you don't know how you feel? So many of us have difficulty not only talking about our emotions but recognizing what they are and expressing them in a safe and healthy manner. Learning to identify and express emotions through our bodies is essential, especially when we feel confined by the thoughts in our heads.

## Moving Our Emotions

According to dance/movement therapist Tal Shafir, "Exploration and practice of new and unfamiliar motor patterns can help [us] experience new unaccustomed feelings."[37] When we move more, we have the potential to feel more. Unlike exercise usually associated with releasing endorphins that boost mood, general movement can bring up uncomfortable, unsettling, and sometimes unpleasant emotions. When we open up our bodies to different ways of moving, we have the potential to release hidden, repressed, or forgotten experiences. These can be joyful and positive, but that is not always the case. That is not a reason to avoid movement. On the contrary, this is a reason to engage in more movement—to fully experience and access your emotions. That being said, it should be done gently and slowly. If as you tap into a greater embodied awareness you experience overwhelming emotions, know that support is available. Resources for additional support are available at the end of this book.

Moving mindfully is very different than exercising, which can be done on autopilot. In fact, there are many instances where people engage in movement as a distraction. How do you know if you are using movement as a distraction? One key sign is that you are ignoring your body. There is a difference between challenging yourself and overriding your body's internal alarm. Movement in all forms should never be used as a punishment. Ideally it is used to support your physical and emotional health. If your movement practice is creating further emotional harm or distress, stop or seek support around it. With great movement comes great responsibility. Even yoga has the potential to trigger emotional overwhelm or anxiety. The smallest, gentlest movement has the potential to open up parts of us that we didn't know were there.

It is possible to use movement to support your emotions. Even for those with little to no experience, movement is a way to reset your emotional compass. It is ideal to practice this and engage your body before feeling overcome by stress, as that will inhibit your ability to be present to your needs in the moment. Movement should not just be seen as a crisis intervention, but as a proactive tool that can actually help manage the emotions before they lead to a crisis. Being body aware is all about utilizing your body's knowledge to assist in the management of your emotions. This requires three steps:

1. **IDENTIFY IT.** Identifying an emotion can be done in two ways: either by bringing awareness to an emotion you are currently experiencing or by first noticing how your body feels and then naming an emotion associated with that feeling. In both cases, it is about identifying what parts of your body connect to and house different emotions. One way you can practice this is through a body scan. Start by revisiting the Movement Rx in chapter 1. As you identify sensations in parts of your body, notice what emotions you associate with them. You can get creative and think about the color, shape, or size of the emotion as well. As you uncover these different emotions and how they exist in your body, I suggest you keep a journal tracking them. Putting them down on paper not only makes them visible but keeps

you out of your head—which means less attention on the mind and more focus on the body.

**2. EXPRESS IT.**   Once you have identified an emotion, find a way to express it through your body. Remember back to my client in chapter 3 who struggled with anxiety. In order to identify where in her body she was feeling her anxiety, Sara placed her hand to her stomach and focused on the rhythm and intensity of the anxiety. This was displayed in intense circling, which morphed into gentle massaging. Expression could be dancing it out or creating a posture or gesture that represents the emotion. Feeling the emotion is only the beginning. A body aware practice means engaging with it, moving it. For individuals who have experience with dance and movement, give yourself the opportunity to dance as the emotion, with the emotion, and in response to it.

**3. SUPPORT IT.**   You might notice the emotion has a specific rhythm about it. Perhaps it's a vibration, a pounding, a swing or sway. Find the rhythm and move with it. Feel free to use music to support this rhythm. Be sure that the music supports the current emotion and not the emotion you wish to feel.

This practice can be done in the comfort of your bedroom or in a bathroom stall at a restaurant while you are out to dinner or on a date. I have encouraged my clients to give themselves permission to use this when they need it, not when it is convenient. Our emotions don't wait for the "right" time to come up. They are always present and when we meet them as they emerge instead of pushing them aside or pretending they don't exist, the fear around expressing them lessens and the ability to access them increases.

This ability to be with and move our emotions brings about a new awareness. When we know what we feel, we are able to differentiate between what is ours and what belongs to others. Have you ever felt responsible for someone else's feelings? Do you find yourself apologizing even though you didn't do anything wrong? Being able to identify our emotions holds us accountable to our own experiences and releases the need to be responsible for others' emotions. Connecting to your emotions and understanding how they feel in your body enables you to set boundaries. Boundaries, while challenging to enforce, when found through the body, permit us to speak our truth unapologetically.

## Creating Boundaries, Setting Limits

Boundaries are a hot topic in the therapy world. There are many definitions floating around. They are essentially limits, both physical and emotional, that when set meet a personal need, or when unmet perpetuate emotional harm and in some instances physical danger.

Boundaries are important because they provide a foundation for self-respect, integrity, and self-worth. Boundaries are more about saying yes to yourself than they are about saying no to others, because when you say yes to everything and everyone, the person you are really saying no to is you.

Sometimes it is helpful to look at what something isn't to understand what it is. What does it look like to have a lack of boundaries? A difficulty setting boundaries in childhood often carries over to adulthood.[38] When we are young and not given boundaries, we don't know how to set them later, and if others try to set them with us, we can have a hard time managing them. A lack of boundaries in the body can show up as invading others' personal space. This can happen one, because we are unaware of our own body in space; two, because we are unable to register how others feel when we invade their space; and three, the other person may be unaware of their own personal boundaries as well. On the other hand, a very rigid, tight body may have very strict boundaries related to fear, control, vulnerability, safety, or harm.

> **BODY AWARE BREAK** Bring your attention to the word *yes*. You may even want to say it out loud and see where it lands in your body. What is your current relationship with this word? Now try bringing your attention to the word *no*. Say it if necessary and again bring awareness to how your body says it nonverbally. Which one feels more familiar? Which feels more accessible?

Growing up I often associated saying no to others as mean. I feared that people wouldn't like me. It was more important that people think of me as kind and nice than it was for me to listen to my own needs. While I have found it difficult to set and even hold boundaries with certain people in my life, using my body to explore this construct has been life-changing. When I began to integrate a body aware lens into noticing and creating boundaries, I was able to see that the boundary was not for others but for me. Not only can we look at the boundaries of our physical being but we can also use sensations that arise in the body when faced with situations that challenge our limits. I have often said to my clients that dance/movement therapy is about learning to compromise without compromising the Self. This to me refers to recognizing your own limits and boundaries so that you have the ability to know who you are and what you need without sacrificing those for the benefit of others.

You might be familiar with the phrases "bend over backwards" and "pushover." These quite literally speak to how we embody a lack of boundaries. It suggests that we not only get pushed around, but that it can feel compromising and uncomfortable. I was seeing a woman in her mid-thirties who was overwhelmed, to say the least. She mentioned that her back gave her a lot of problems and it was often sore. While this wasn't the primary reason she came to therapy, it was important for me to know so that as we moved together I knew what parts of her body might be extra sensitive. Since her back was particularly sore this day, I invited her to pay attention to it and listen to what it needed.

She began in Child's Pose, perched on her shins with her chest resting on her upper thighs, gently stretching her arms out in front of her, lowering her head to the floor and breathing into her back. Without prompting she started to talk about when she was a kid, dancing and doing backbends. I asked her if she still did those, to which she said no. But then she began to talk about why she doesn't do them. "I don't dance anymore," she said. "I don't really have time for myself since I had a family." She went on to explain that she did everything for them and whether she wanted to or not it was the role that was assumed. "I've always been one to bend over backwards." This stopped me in my tracks. I asked her, "Do you think your sore back has anything to do accommodating others?" She paused, her eyes widened, and she said, "I never thought about it in that way, but ever since I can remember I have overextended myself. Physically I push beyond my limits, I have always been hyper-flexible, and I never know where to stop."

Of course a sore back happens for many different reasons, but for her it became a metaphor for her inability to set limits for herself and others. It was a way for us to explore how she could create healthy boundaries and learn to compromise without sacrificing her own physical and emotional safety.

> **BODY AWARE BREAK** Sit with your back against the wall. Bring into your awareness all the ways your body is touching the wall. Now notice the spaces between your body and the wall—for example, the curve of your neck and lower back. Allow yourself to push gently into the wall and notice how it feels when you ease the pressure. Oscillate between pushing into the wall and leaning away from the wall. This movement doesn't have to be big—in fact, the smaller the better.

Dance/movement therapist and counselor Dee Wagner says, "When I push into what is Not-Me, I find Me."[39] In other words, when we explore our boundaries and limits we are able to identify who we are and what it is we need. Wagner invites people to do this with a partner, but I find this quote resonates with the above experience. When you push into the wall, you may feel the boundaries of where you end and the wall begins. You can physically feel your body's boundaries. You can use the wall for support and as a safe way to explore your own limits. Can you internalize those as you lean away from the wall? How do you uphold those limits and enforce that boundary? This concept of pushing and pulling or playing with pressure is something I find to be invaluable when connecting to my own desire to give in or my ability to stand firm.

So what does setting limits look like from a body aware perspective? It begins with recognizing how boundaries or lack thereof impact your movement. Do you curl up or shrink so as not to be visible? Does your body overcompensate and exude defensiveness? Noticing how our bodies react to limits in our environment is vital to harnessing our own ability to set boundaries in order to meet our own needs. Three steps you can take to prime your body for setting limits are:

1. **ACCESS YOUR SPINE.**   If you recall the Head-Tail Connectivity, this is where we connect to our self-awareness. When we bring attention and focus to the spine, this provides an opportunity to check in with ourselves.[40] When we provide time to recognize who we are, what we feel, and what we need, we are better equipped to know what limits need to be set. You can access your spine by bringing attention to the vertical—lifting your upper body or shifting your posture.

2. **MANIPULATE THE SPINE.**   I don't mean through chiropractic or physical therapy. I mean move your spine in unconventional ways, safely of course. Your spine has curves, and it allows you to spiral and twist. Allow your spine to gently curve, swivel, spiral, and twist. You may try rounding or arching your back, tilting your shoulders side to side, or gently reaching both arms to either side as you look behind you. You can try isolating different parts of your spine, moving your rib cage or lower back. This I believe is what paves the way for embodied resilience, which will be discussed further in chapter 8.

3. **PUSH, PULL, AND REACH.**   Try on these three movements. I encourage you to use props and other items in your environment to activate or support these movements. Never underestimate the use of a wall; lean on it, push into it, like in the body aware break above. Notice what you feel in your body with regard to placing boundaries on and around you. The idea is to be able to push without being pushed around, pull without being dragged, and reach for your own needs and goals—not just to help others. Through these interventions, you can begin to identify how it feels when others place limits on you, notice how it feels when you minimize your own needs, and

practice implementing limits by learning to access them initially through the body.

—

Up to this point, this chapter has provided insight into how current movement influences thoughts and behaviors. There is another important piece to changing our thoughts with regard to movement and that is proactively and intentionally using movement to move the mind. Now, we'll focus on mindfully incorporating movement into your everyday life. Here are some additional movement prescriptions that can help support you on your journey to becoming body aware.

## Inviting Movement into Your Day

If you are still hesitant or unsure of how to add movement into your day, that is okay. For those of you who are still feeling compelled to think your way out, you can try journaling with a twist. I created the Body Awareness for Mental Health Journal when I realized that many people fell into this category. This will help you begin to connect the dots between what you feel and how it influences your mind. I suggest journaling at the beginning or end of the day, and limiting distractions in order to practice listening to your body. Try this once or twice a week and build from there.

---

## Body Awareness for Mental Health Journal Prompts

Something I feel in my body is _____.

This impacts my mental health because _____.

Actions I will take to address this are _____.

---

Here's an example of a filled-in journal entry:

---

## Body Awareness for Mental Health Journal Prompts

Something I feel in my body is *tension in my shoulders*.

This impacts my mental health because *this causes pain, which makes me irritable*.

Actions I will take to address this are *rolling my shoulders throughout the day*.

---

If journaling isn't quite your cup of tea, then consider jumping right into the body. Set reminders (write a note or set an alarm on your phone) that invite you to take movement breaks throughout the day. Here are thirty movement prompts to get you started.

**30 MOVEMENT PROMPTS TO GET YOU OUT OF YOUR HEAD AND INTO YOUR BODY**

1. Notice your breath.

2. Take a breath.

3. Stretch your arms.

4. Put your feet on the floor.

5. Give yourself a hug.

6. Wiggle your fingers.

7. Stomp your feet.

8. Shake your hands.

9. Rub your hands together.

10. Tap or pat your legs.

11. Have an impromptu dance party.

12. Play "head, shoulders, knees, and toes."

13. Do the twist.

14. Do the floss!

15. Jump 5 times.

16. Tap each finger to your thumb.

17. Slow down your movement

18. Write with your nondominant hand.

19. Take up space with your body.

20. Tap your fingers over your face.

21. Identify 3 things you can see.

22. Move to a different part of the room.

23. Sing a song.

24. Express an emotion without words.

25. Yawn.

26. Interlace your fingers and squeeze.

27. Raise and lower your shoulders.

28. Shake your body.

29. March in place.

30. Shift your posture.

These are simply suggestions meant to help you prioritize movement, getting you out of your head and into your body. It is important to organically and authentically implement these as forcing them will only be counterproductive. Be aware of any tendencies to immerse yourself in this new practice, as that can be a pattern in itself. Remember, it's not just about the movement itself, but your intention and focus. Bonnie Bainbridge Cohen says, "It's very important when you do a movement that your attention (which is what is stimulating you) and your intent (which is what you want to do in relation to that stimulation) align up with the movement that you're doing."[41] We don't want to perpetuate autopilot, but create awareness around our habits and invite in new ways of moving and being.

## Starting Your Day off on the Right (or Left) Foot

You know the old saying, "got up on the wrong side of the bed"? This suggests that our mood is connected to how we feel when we wake up, even before we physically get up. Moving your body in certain ways allows your mind to wake up and show up for the day before you even get out of bed.

**BREATHE.** You know that moment when you first become aware that you are waking up? Your eyes aren't even open yet, but you just know that you're not going back to sleep. This is when you want to focus on your breath. Notice it, invite it into your body, and allow it to take up space wherever possible. Pay attention to where you first feel it in your body. Beginning with where you feel it, imagine sending it to other parts of your body. Infuse your body with your breath, letting it wash over you from the top of your head to the tips of your toes. I find it helpful to add imagery, like waves in the ocean or a cool breeze, as the breath washes over and through you.

**STRETCH OUT.** When I wake up I'm usually in the fetal position with the blanket right up to my face, arms and hands tightly pulled into my chest. My body is small, bound, and rigid. This is not the way I want to get up and out. After I have lubricated my body with my breath, I reach into the four corners of my bed. I slowly transition to my back as I reach my feet to the bottom corners and my hands to the top corners. I understand that space may still be limited due to significant others or furry friends. Do your best to stretch out and embody the space you want to take up in your day, in your life. One of my fondest memories from when both of my children were infants was going into their room in the morning, unswaddling them, and watching them take their first stretch of the day. Like clockwork, it felt to me as if the body was preparing to take on the day and open itself and the mind to new experiences. I see this mirrored in the way my dogs wake up as well—stretching, rolling, and shaking off a deep sleep in order to take on the day.

**PLANT YOUR FEET.** By now you are probably toying with the idea of getting out of bed. This is when you want to be intentional with your grounding and balance. If you are still not quite ready to get up, bring your knees up and place your feet on the bed. Allow your pelvis to shift or rock. Engage your spine. Breathe. If you are ready to get out of bed, roll to your side and slowly swing your feet around toward the floor. Before you stand, take time to plant your feet on the ground. Feel the texture of the floor beneath you. Give yourself an opportunity to find your connection to the floor as you slowly come to standing. This is your metaphor for standing on your own two feet in the world. Stake your claim as you stand up and lengthen through your spine.

**REACH UP AND OUT.**  Now allow your body to reach into the space above you. This looks different for everyone. It might be your chin looking up to the ceiling, or your arms reaching to the sky. Next, explore the space below your hips. Can you reach down or even let your hands make contact with your thighs and gently trace them along your legs? Play in this space until you feel your spine is waking up. Lastly, reach your arms across your body, giving yourself a hug and then spread your arms out, reaching to either side of the room. Now you are ready to move forward, walking into your day with intention and awareness.

This routine can be modified based on your physical abilities. You can also assist someone with this routine if they cannot do this safely on their own. In chapter 9, I'll further discuss diversity and accessibility in movement practices. Keep in mind that it is just as important to end your day with movement. If you are prone to a fast-paced day, it is necessary to slow yourself down in order to ease yourself into rest and sleep. Pay attention to how you are moving right before bed and make sure it is supporting the recharge you need at the end of the day. This routine can be used to ease yourself into bedtime as well. You may find it helpful to reverse the order, ending with movement designed to connect to the Self—letting go of the activities and interactions from the day and coming back home to your mind and body.

## Opportunities for Movement Are Everywhere

I understand that movement doesn't always feel possible, especially when life has other plans. The idea isn't to bring movement to you, it is about bringing yourself to movement. Here are some other ways I invite movement into my day, especially when I don't have time or space to move freely.

DRIVING.    If you are anything like me, you spend a large portion of your day driving. I actually love driving, but that doesn't always mean I am doing it mindfully. A couple ways I have used driving to increase my emotional miles per gallon (more on this in chapter 8) is by accessing my breath at a red light. When I am forced to stop in my car, I use it as an opportunity to start accessing my body. I breathe into my abdomen and feel my back widen into the seat as I take a deep cleansing breath—in through my nose and out through my mouth, exhaling slightly longer than my inhale. This signals the "rest and digest" reflex by activating the vagus nerve, the longest and most complex cranial nerve responsible for sending out information from the brain's surface throughout the body. Central to Polyvagal Theory, the vagus nerve essentially balances the nervous system.[42] More information can be found in the resource section at the end of the book.

I also use my time in the car to shift my pacing. If I am in a hurry I tend to be heavier on the accelerator, as opposed to when I am fatigued or relaxed. Drawing my attention to this pattern allows me to accelerate on my own time not because of an external need to get somewhere. Notice how much your driving habits coincide with your emotional state. Let's just say there is a reason it's called "road rage."

SINGING.    You don't have to be a good singer to do this one. Whether it is in the car, kitchen, or shower, practice belting out a good tune. Not only can singing support emotional expression but it can also help connect you to your breath. This reinforces the earlier idea that movement enhances vocal support.

COOKING.    I can't say I practice this one as often as I'd like, but this is a great opportunity to use your body. Play some music in the background and move your way around the kitchen as you chop, slice, and peel. Pay attention to the aromas and sounds as you prepare your meal. This may even allow you to enjoy your food more as you connect to the experience and not just the end result.

## Next Steps

So you are prioritizing movement, becoming more aware of how and when to implement it into your life, but you may be wondering *what's next?* Remember in part 1 how I spoke about increasing your movement repertoire, also known as your movement vocabulary? The next step is learning to expand your movement vocabulary. This is the key to managing your emotions. We will explore how increasing your range of movement and building your vocabulary supports your emotional capacity and tolerance to stressors. You can tolerate your emotional load by relying on your body to foster emotional regulation. Let's fly!

## Move Your Body, Move Your Mind in Motion

When Ronnie came to me, she made it clear that she loved to dance but lacked any motivation to move at all. Concerned with her weight and wanting to be more physically active, she was hoping to uncover the reason behind this lack of motivation and find a gentle way to start moving again.

I simply asked Ronnie to move around the studio, and she began walking with purpose at a quick tempo. There wasn't a lot of freedom in her torso, and her upper body was rather bound. I asked her how this felt, and she replied that it was just like her to push through and move through things quickly. She stopped . . . unable to move forward any more. So I invited her to move in another direction. She began walking backward, which to her surprise felt comfortable. She said, "I feel like I can trust myself." She walked through the space, slightly looking over her shoulder so as not to bump into anything, but able to trust that her body would guide her. I invited her to move sideways. Ronnie began sidestepping and then her shoulder started to roll. I asked her to comment on what that felt like. Instantly she said, "Creative."

This began a conversation on how she was shamed for being the creative one in the family and that after her dad's death when she was a child, her creative side was suppressed. She walked over to the ballet barre, where she began stretching her back, pulling gently on the barre with her feet planted firmly. She started walking her body into the barre and back out, stretching her arms out in front of her. Back and forth she walked, holding onto the barre. I pointed out that she was walking forward. She smirked and said, "I know." I asked why that was. Ronnie said, "I have support." So she realized that she could move forward in her life if she had a supportive team. I asked if she was ready to try walking forward away from the barre, and hesitantly she said yes. She began walking forward but on a diagonal, side to side, rolling her shoulder as she stepped. When asked to reflect, Ronnie said, "I can move forward if I have my creativity with me."

## MOVEMENT RX: MOVE YOUR BODY, SHIFT YOUR MIND

*Directions:*  Identify how you are feeling emotionally at this moment.

Begin to invite in some simple movements. Take some deep breaths, walk around your house or office, stretch your body to activate your muscles, have an impromptu dance party, or do all of the above. Feel free to reference the movement prompts from earlier in this chapter.

Mindfully engage in this movement experience for two to three minutes.

Take a moment to check back in with your mood. Did moving your body shift your mood in any way? If so, how?

*Dosage:*  Use when attempting to manage challenging emotions.

*Side Effects:*  Enhanced ability to regulate emotions.

## TAKEAWAYS

* We must feel our way through in order to then think our way out.

* Movement is an extension of the Self.

* A change in movement impacts who we are.

* Meet the body where it is in order to guide the mind where you want it to go.

* When you feel stuck emotionally, you always have the option to move physically.

# 5

## PLANES ARE NOT
## JUST FOR FLYING

*Time and space are not conditions of existence;*
*time and space are models of thinking.*
—ALBERT EINSTEIN

## Charting the Course

Growing up as a dancer, I was very aware of how to move around the dance floor. Marking routines, making sure to find the X on the stage in order to be in the right place, and moving into different formations was familiar. While movement naturally occurs in planes, it didn't occur to me that I could intentionally move my own body in these dimensional planes as well until I began to learn modern dance technique in my high school dance program. It was there that I got exposed to the techniques and teachings of Westernized modern dance, which was born out of a need for the body to rebel against the strictures of ballet. Modern dancers understand that the body needs to express itself through free movement.

**BODY AWARE BREAK** Bring attention to your body. Tense your muscles as much as possible. Notice what this feels like. Now relax those same muscles. This illustrates what the modern dance world was looking to experience through movement: a sense of liberation and embodied freedom.

This not only changed my perception of dance but marked the beginning of my own journey into body awareness through movement. From rolling around on the floor, spiraling, contracting and releasing, and learning the basics of Bartenieff's fundamentals, I began to feel more alive in my body than ever before. Little did I know this would lay the groundwork for my career.

Fast-forward to graduate school where I was formally introduced to Laban Movement Analysis (LMA), a systemic way to quantify and qualify movement. Being immersed in Laban's work was interesting, to say the least. Honestly, his framework was very confusing to me, and the intricate system he created never really seemed to fit my body. I never questioned it, since early academic conditioning taught me to believe that anything could be learned in order to get an A. Once I graduated I was happy to detach from LMA, since I didn't understand how it would directly help my clients, who at the time were older adults living with cognitive impairments mostly due to dementia. I found myself going back to Bartenieff's fundamentals of connectivity, previously discussed in chapter 4, realizing that it was necessary to foster connection in the body to create connection to me and other group participants. Also, I was looking for ways to literally move the body in an attempt to create opportunities for discussion and processing.

At the same time I struggled to find my own flow in my groups. I so often followed the structure of dance/movement therapists I had studied in school, but that lacked authenticity and creativity. I remember trying to find a ritual with which to begin and end my groups. Again, trying on others' rituals only added to the frustration, until one day I revisited LMA. I remembered back to the only part of LMA that really made sense to my body: Laban's One-Dimensional or Defense Scale.[1] This is "built around the axes of the three dimensions of the body: length, width, and depth, and their corresponding axes in space of the kinesphere: vertical, horizontal, and sagittal."[2] Keeping in mind that I was working with people who were non-dancers, older adults, and living with compromised cognition, I broke it down into very basic movements:

**Vertical plane:** Reaching up and down

**Horizontal plane:** Reaching across and to the sides

**Sagittal plane:** Reaching forward and backward[3]

I decided to start every group with this adapted dimensional scale, inviting the participants to reach up and down, across and out, and forward and back. For the most part, this was done seated, which obviously influenced the range of motion in the sagittal plane. I embodied these directions myself, but what I witnessed in the groups went beyond my wildest dreams.

Much like the cases I had studied in school, when participants engaged in the vertical plane they awakened their core self, which housed their identity, thoughts, beliefs, and values. This was evidenced not only by the developmental movement patterns they were exhibiting and accessing but also through verbal feedback in conjunction with the movements, such as "I am here," "I see the sky," and "I am reaching to the heavens." When they engaged in the horizontal plane, they reinforced connection to core self as they wrapped their arms around their torsos, often accompanied by the words "I love me" as they connected to others in the group, literally reaching out to say hello and shake a hand. It is a beautiful sight to see people introduce themselves authentically and unapologetically. Lastly, the sagittal plane supported action and interaction with their surroundings. This was illustrated in how they moved toward the center of the circle and retreated back to their chairs as if to signal "this is me moving into the world and coming back safely to myself."

This became our opening and closing ritual. Through basic embodied dimensions, we were able to connect the mind and body and unleash cognitive potential through movement. I finally found a routine that felt authentic to me and validating to the group participants.

Bessel van der Kolk says, "You can be fully in charge of your life, but only if you can acknowledge the reality of your body, in all its visceral dimensions."[4] Bringing this modified scale to my older adult clients gave them agency, motivation, and orientation. As van der Kolk says, it enabled them to be in charge. Experiencing their bodies through these dimensions allowed them to reclaim or even relearn developmental patterns that had been neglected. I recall this dialogue from one group:

> Me: "Good morning everyone! Let's begin. Join me as we explore our planes!"

> Participant: "Are we flying somewhere?"

> Me: "Ah, good question! Planes aren't just for flying."

Ironically, these planes took us places. They enabled us to travel through our imaginations, creating visceral experiences and making dynamic connections along the way.

Years later, as I began working in private practice with younger clients and individuals not living with dementia, I explored using these planes as a means of assessing and observing a client's connection to the Self, to others, and to their environment. Using LMA as a jumping-off point and in an effort to make these concepts accessible and digestible to non-movers, this was how I broke them down. The vertical reinforced connection to core self, as it brought people through their core in an attempt to access support and mobility in the spine. The horizontal reinforced value and self-worth, as suggested in "I love me" and the need, ability, and/or willingness to connect to others. Meanwhile, the sagittal suggested moving through their environment and taking action.

As I brought clients through these planes, I would invite them to consider which felt familiar, comfortable, or accessible. We would also notice which ones felt inaccessible, and I found that these all mirrored the very issues that brought them to therapy. Picture a client who feels like a prisoner at her high-pressure job and is experiencing burnout. She is familiar with the "go-go-go" forward movement in the sagittal plane. Another client struggling with her self-esteem and body image throws herself into relationships for validation and finds familiarity in the horizontal plane. And lastly the client who is struggling to move forward into adulthood finds it comforting to explore connection to the Self in the vertical plane. These are not my assumptions or judgments, but actual feedback from clients as they experienced what it was like to move through these dimensions and metaphorically through life.

Interestingly, while less familiar dimensions were often uncomfortable, there were plenty of times when clients felt pleasure and recuperation when accessing these unfamiliar planes. I recall a time working with a client who had taken over the family business and it had consumed her to the point where, in her words, she "needed an assistant just to make sure she took bathroom breaks." When I invited her to explore the sagittal plane, she found it very familiar, particularly the forward motion. When I asked her to move backward, she admitted that at first it seemed counterproductive and not in line with her work ethic to push forward and jump into the next project. What she found as she explored it more was that it was exactly what she was looking for. Moving backward allowed her to step back, relax, and take time for herself, something she never allowed herself to do.

Let me be clear that these planes aren't so cut and dried. As I mentioned before, it is up to each individual as to how they embody and experience them. While there are often common themes that come up, it is not about me assuming or assigning meaning, but rather letting the client infer what it brings up for them. The beautiful part is that everyone moves in these dimensions, and when we explore them without automatically assigning meaning or directing the movement in a particular manner, we can own our experience and find agency to do something with the information.

You can access these too! And what's more, you can learn to expand your current affinity toward a plane and explore the other dimensions to create a balanced body and psyche.

We'll begin by exploring each plane and diving into the ways they can help you identify your current mindset and embrace new possibilities.

**BODY AWARE BREAK** If you are able to, stand up with your feet firmly planted on the floor. Feel free to adapt this to your needs and abilities. This can be done in a chair as well. Starting in an upright position, lifting through your spine, begin to reach your arms into the space above your head. Slowly bring your arms down and reach into the space below your knees. Repeat this pattern with intention three times.

Now wrap your arms around your upper body as if to give yourself an embrace. Slowly open your arms and reach out to either side. Repeat this pattern with intention three times.

Finally, reach your arms into the space in front of you, allowing them to pull you into a forward motion. Slowly bring your arms back and allow your body to move in a backward direction. Repeat this pattern with intention three times.

Take a few minutes to identify overall which plane (vertical, horizontal, sagittal) felt most familiar or accessible and which one felt uncomfortable or the most unpleasant. Next take a few moments to identify which particular direction (up/down, across/open, forward/backward) in those planes felt most familiar or accessible and which one felt uncomfortable or the most unpleasant.

Hopefully this experience gives you some insight into your preferred movement habits. Notice for yourself which ones feel more accessible and which ones do not. While you can use these dimensions to reinforce the areas of your life that are connected, you can engage the less familiar ones to strengthen those connections that need extra support. Or like the example of my client, below, you can explore them to find moments of recuperation and recovery.

Haley entered my studio in an oversized sweatshirt and baggy pants. Her hair was covering her eyes and her gaze was mostly on the floor. She held her arms around her upper body and exhibited a slouched posture. I felt a lack of presence as exhibited in her sunken core and predicted that in order to bring that into the room, she needed to explore the vertical plane.

I invited Haley to explore the space above her head. She slowly began to reach her arms above her shoulders as if she were going to touch the ceiling. The movement was confined to her arms and there was little to no activation in her torso. I then invited her to reach into the space below her knees. She slowly leaned down toward her feet and began to engage her spine and core muscles. We played in this vertical movement for quite some time, oscillating between the two polarities. Her torso and chest engaged a little more each time she reached into the opposing directions. On the last time, her posture shifted and remained lifted, her eyes made contact with mine, and her arms relaxed by her sides. We looked at each other. I asked her to describe what happened and what she felt. She said that for the first time in years she felt connected to her body, something that she spent most of her time intentionally avoiding.

Engaging in these planes is easier for some than others. One person may have an immediate epiphany, while another may need to revisit it over and over again before the slightest shift takes place. It is important to prioritize practicing these planes because, as we know, practice makes habit. The more you practice engaging in unfamiliar patterns, the more familiar they become—ultimately creating new patterns of thought and behavior.

## Getting Ready for Departure

Do you identify with any of these situations?

- You are always on the go, never stopping, only to crash at the end of the day.
- You only participate in high-intensity exercise and cannot stand the thought of meditation or yoga.
- You procrastinate or have difficulty getting motivated.
- You see the world as "all or nothing" and find it challenging to embrace the in-between.

These mindsets are all reinforced by movement habits and patterns. As mentioned in the last chapter, they are adaptable. However, they cannot be changed without understanding and acknowledging how they exist in your body. You have to identify your place of departure before you can choose your destination.

Looking at how these three planes reinforce your current flight pattern is the best place to start. Keep in mind that there are many ways in which these are embodied. Let me break down some of the ways they have come up in my own life as well as in those of my clients.

VERTICAL. This plane is where I find my grounding and center. When I feel overwhelmed by my thoughts and need to reconnect to my body I can rely on this plane to bring me back home to my body. Clients have verbalized that this plane allows them to connect to a higher power as they reach toward the heavens or find connection to the Earth with their feet planted on the ground as they reach down. For some clients this is a less desirable plane that brings up self-doubt, low self-esteem, and body image issues. It is difficult for some individuals to be with and in their body so the ability to access the vertical plane is challenging, but rewarding in the end.

HORIZONTAL. This is where I can bring myself into connection with others. When I am in need of support, advocating for my needs, and encouraging myself to ask for help, I go to this plane. It allows me to access the sense of self I feel in the vertical and share it with my loved ones. For many clients this plane is about acknowledging vulnerability and trust. Exploring how trust is embodied and how a lack of trust shows up in the ability to extend and reach out to others in a time of need. There can be safety and comfort in embracing one's own body. As we reach out to either side and open the chest, our hearts are exposed, leading to a sense of openness that, for example, can welcome in feelings of love or fear of getting hurt.

SAGITTAL. This is where I go when I need to take action or take a step back to reevaluate or assess a situation. Clients have expressed this plane as housing feelings around confrontation as they move toward someone or backing down as they move away. Moving forward can suggest searching, pushing through, or going into the unknown, whereas moving backward can feel like a setback, running from the past, or retracing old steps.

I cannot stress enough that there is no "right" way to feel in each plane. Each direction is an opportunity to create metaphors through movement. These are merely examples of what I have experienced in my work, personally and professionally. Keep in mind that things like personal experience, culture, and geography will influence how these planes are interpreted. I encourage you to explore these planes and see what themes and metaphors come up for you.

As addressed in part I, movement patterns and habits are not just the directions in which we move but the qualities of the movement itself. Looking at how you move and the nuances of your movements, in addition to which qualities you are drawn to, has the ability to take you to new heights of awareness and understanding with regard to how your movement impacts your mood and mental health.

## Soaring to New Heights

Realizing how beneficial exploring these planes was with my clients, I revisited other LMA components. I remembered learning about motion factors Laban identified as time, space, weight, and flow, which you'll learn more about below.[5]

When I brought this work to my clients in private practice, we initially explored polarities of each element. For example, taking up as much space as possible versus making my body as small as I can helps me identify which feels more accessible and comfortable in my body. Eventually we entertained the idea of moving on a spectrum to facilitate a greater range of motion that corresponds to more possibilities and options in how I manage daily stressors. The "all or nothing" mindset, also known as dichotomous thinking, was challenged when clients were encouraged to explore the gray area in between.

With regard to exploring movement qualities, we are going to focus on space, time, and weight, as these are the common ones identified in my private practice. Before I break down each one, these are the three steps we are going to focus on:

1. Identify your polarities.

2. Embody each polarity.

3. Practice moving between polarities, looking at the spectrum of movement.

Here are some ideas of polarities to get you started:

| SPACE | TIME | WEIGHT |
|---|---|---|
| Big/little | Fast/slow | Heavy/light |
| Near/far | Steady/syncopated | Pressure/release |
| Narrow/wide | On-time/delayed | Focused/scattered |

Give yourself two to three minutes to engage in each polarity before attempting to move between them.

Now let's highlight some metaphors for each quality:

| SPACE | TIME | WEIGHT |
|---|---|---|
| Distance | Efficiency | Body |
| Personal boundaries | Motivation | Responsibility |
| Freedom | Responsiveness | Focus |

Here are some questions for reflection following this experience:

**SPACE**

*How does space show up in my life?*

*Do I need a lot of personal space?*

*What are my cultural implications of space?*

*Am I allowed to take up space?*

*Do I like to take up space, or do I make myself small and invisible?*

*What happens when I don't have enough space or feel confined?*

**TIME**

*Am I conscious of time?*

*Do I have time?*

*Is my time my own, or do I feel like I am on someone else's time?*

*Do I procrastinate?*

*Am I early or on time?*

*Am I always on the go, or do I give myself opportunities to slow down?*

**WEIGHT**

*Do I feel pressured?*

*How does stress show up in my body?*

*Do I have difficulty being direct with people?*

*Do I space out or find it difficult to be present?*

*Am I able to focus, or do I get easily distracted?*

By understanding and becoming aware of which motion factors feel most familiar, you can continue to identify your current movement profile and increase it as more movement becomes possible and tolerable. As clients were able to tolerate different movement, they noticed that their ability to tolerate stressors was also increasing. A greater range in movement correlated to a greater range of emotional capacity.

## More Room in the Cabin

Who doesn't wish they had more legroom or overhead space on an airplane? This image is a great metaphor for the inability to manage our stress when we lack space to breathe and move. Our emotional capacity is influenced by our physical ability to expand. Capacity can mean the maximum amount something can contain and also the ability or power to do, experience, or understand something. Both of these definitions are important because we are going to uncover how tapping into your internal "legroom" helps support your emotional capacity.

There is a connection between our physical capacity and how much emotional baggage we can carry on. Amy Cuddy, social psychologist and best-selling author, says, "Expanding your body expands your mind."[6] We can increase our emotional capacity through movement. Dan Siegel, executive director of the Mindsight Institute, says that each person has a "window of tolerance,"[7] a varying degree of emotional arousal that can be endured without totally derailing a person's ability to function. Behavior and cognition are disrupted when a person moves outside the boundaries of that "window." Interestingly enough, at each end of the arousal spectrum, individuals experience responses in the body such as an increased heart rate and respiration due to hyper-arousal or a decrease in heart rate and respiration due to hypo-arousal. In hyper-arousal the focus is on energy consumption, while in hypo-arousal the focus is on energy conservation. A person will experience either a heightened state of alertness or a shutting down. In both cases the clear path to getting back inside the window of tolerance as well as expanding that window is through movement.

Somatic body-based interventions like mindfulness, meditation, yoga, and breathwork are just a few examples of what mental health specialists might recommend in order for a person to return to optimal functioning. While these are beneficial, the interventions alone are not enough. We must look at how they are introduced and implemented. It is not just about the exercise alone. It is about the execution.

Let's begin by looking at your breath as a way to measure and alter your internal capacity. Notice your breath right now. Where do you feel it? I'm guessing most of you reading this will identify it in your chest. What if I told you that by moving your breath into the belly you could actually support your ability to regulate your emotions? When your breath resides in your chest as opposed to your abdomen, it limits your ability to regulate your nervous system. When we begin to challenge how we breathe, we can identify places in the body that can access breath. When we increase our ability to breathe, we inevitably create more space in the body, and making space in the body creates space in the mind. We can create space in the body to make room to process emotions and feelings.

Breath becomes the current that flows through the body, creating opportunities for increased flexibility. Flexibility is more than a perfect split or yoga pose. It is about mobility, adaptability, fluidity, and transition within movement in all forms within the body. The more we are able to move and create flexible bodies, the more flexible we can be in our minds. We can think in the moment, focus, be more productive, make decisions, and problem solve. Some people are flexible in their minds. Some people are flexible in their bodies. The goal is to be someone who is both. Flexibility of the body can correlate to flexibility of the mind, which means supporting the ability to think in the moment and cope with or manage emotions in crisis or periods of stress.

I used to suffer from horrible "white-coat syndrome," otherwise known as fear of doctors. No matter how much I warned the medical staff and assured them my high blood pressure was my frantic nervous system, I would undoubtedly get the advice to "just take some deep breaths." To say that was less than helpful would be an understatement. One day in a doctor's office, waiting for what seemed like a lifetime, I decided to take matters into my own hands. I hopped off the examination table and rather than "calming down," I matched the rhythm inside my body. I matched the intense pounding in my chest with a jump, repeating it until I could feel the pounding lessen. While my heart rate was still elevated, I could literally feel the energy shift. I slowed down the jumping and bounced my knees, noticing that I was finally able to access my breath. The breath was no longer frozen in my shoulders but was moving its way down toward my belly. My body began to gently sway. I stood up tall, took a deep breath in through my nose and exhaled out my mouth. I stretched my arms over my head and let out a huge sigh. I sat back down and waited for the doctor. For perhaps the first time since the days of going to my pediatrician, my blood pressure reading was normal. Rather than going through the motions, I met my body where it was in its stress response. Only then was I able to introduce calmer rhythms to regulate my nervous system and come back to my window of tolerance.

Ever since I can remember I have used a garage door as a metaphor for regulating emotions. Even though not everyone has a garage door in real life, most of us know what it is and how it works: a typically mechanized device powered by a remote that controls how the door opens, closes, or remains somewhere in between. Prior to our work, my clients tended to either keep their emotional garage doors tightly sealed, needing massive amounts of oil to grease the hinges, or wide open, allowing all of the outside elements to come spilling in—including a random rodent or bird who takes up residence without permission. I tell my clients that the tools and resources they will gain from dance/movement therapy represent a remote control that allows them to open and close the door as needed. The idea sounds good in theory, but the thought of moving the door is frightening. Through exploration of body boundaries, personal space, and basic body awareness, as well as mindful movement and mindfulness, clients begin to explore what it feels like to regulate their own doors as they learn to regulate their emotions.

When we actively engage the body in this process, the magic unfolds. The body becomes the greatest untapped resource to manage and cope with the overwhelming arousal that sends people beyond their own limits. It brings them back from an experience that often catches people off-guard and leaves them drowning in a sea of panic or existential exhaustion.

Not only is movement the way back inside the window, but it is the best way to increase the size of the window. I once had a client say, "Don't open the window if you can't close it." So often, clients are fearful that the therapist will push them too far, uncover a deep secret, or know more about them than they know about themselves. It is not my responsibility to close the window. It is my job to empower the client and arm them with the tools to monitor their own window. It is my ethical duty to create a safe space in which the client can explore and challenge the boundaries of the window and find a way back inside.

## Preparing for Arrival

Movement not only prepares us to take off and adjust our flight plan, but it also assists in transitioning through turbulence. Transition is another big theme that comes up in many of my client sessions. Whether it is a college student transitioning to adulthood, an older adult maneuvering through retirement, or managing a midlife crisis, life is about transition. This can be a struggle for even the most seasoned therapist as life is filled with uncertainty, and how we embody transition is yet another way to support our mental health through welcome or unwarranted change.

**BODY AWARE BREAK** Choose two points in a room. We'll call one place point A and the other point B. Starting at point A, I want you to get to point B as efficiently as possible. Now go back the same way you did to get there. Try that a couple of times to get a good feel for the experience. Now starting at point A again, go to point B as *in*efficiently as possible. Travel back. Do this a few times to solidify the experience. Which one felt more familiar with regard to how you transition from one thing to the next? Which one do you wish you could experience more often?

Transition is moving, passing through, or changing from one thing to another. Many people struggle with transition. They either want to get to the destination as quickly as possible or have trouble initiating the transition altogether. It is difficult and often uncomfortable to be in transition. You may be familiar with the phrase "it's the journey, not the destination," or "it's the process, not the product." Movement has a wonderful way of allowing us to explore the journey, to be in process.

Try this: Create two different postures in your body and mindfully transition from one to the other and back. What do you notice from beginning to end? Does your ability to transition get easier? Is it more tolerable? This, like all other body aware experiences, takes practice. If you are having a hard time making a decision or moving from one phase to another, challenge the way your body supports or resists it.

I am reminded of that high school yet again. With a student body of four thousand, the hallways were always jam-packed and the passing periods were up to ten minutes long to accommodate for the travel between buildings. Thinking back, I can still feel my body tensing up in preparation for the sprint after the bell rang. This says a lot about me and my conditioning to time. I'm definitely one of those people who feels like being early is on time and being on time is late. It drives me crazy knowing that I am running behind. That was until I adopted a body aware perspective with regard to how I transition that not only empowers me to accept limitations but also allows me to stay connected when things are out of my control. Whether I am on time or running late, it has been so important for me to refocus and bring awareness to my body. A body aware perspective on transition entails:

**PAYING ATTENTION TO YOUR BODY.** This is your reminder to bring awareness to those sensations and signals that your body is expressing. This is your compass guiding you to the parts that need attention.

**PARTICIPATING IN MINDFUL MOVEMENT TO CONNECT TO THE PRESENT MOMENT.** Focus on how your body is moving. Turn off autopilot and move with awareness and intention.

**INTENTIONALLY SLOWING DOWN TO DO MORE.** This is a tricky one as you may be conditioned to think that slowing down means getting less done or being lazy. Slowing down your movements allows mastery and agency to come into focus. When you have the ability to focus on a task, you can actually get more done. It is quality over quantity. Keep in mind, the amount of time may be the same, but the quality changes.

## Enjoy Your Stay

Wherever you are traveling on this journey to becoming body aware, take time to acknowledge the victories along the way. You are bound to have delays and even cancellations—meaning you will fall into old habits. It is how you move through them that is the key to making permanent change. Letting go of judgments and being curious about your patterning is an important part of this voyage—not to mention the key to unlocking your greatest potential.

## Planes Aren't Just for Flying in Motion

Jess, a twenty-eight-year-old woman, came to dance/movement therapy because she reported being out of touch with herself: her needs, wants, and values. This was a part she desperately wanted to connect to because she felt it was impacting her ability to trust herself and let go of others' expectations and approval. She explained that she had spent most of her adult life meeting others' demands and overlooking her own needs. And much of her childhood was spent caring for her siblings and being "a good daughter."

I invited her to simply move through the studio, letting her body do what it needed in the moment. Naturally, she began to explore different planes: reaching up, down, across her body, and opening her arms to the side. I asked her to find a movement (pose, gesture, etc.) that represented her "true self."

With her eyes closed, Jess took on this pose of a large X-like shape, standing upright with her feet planted firmly on the ground and her arms reaching up over her head. Her torso expanded as her shoulders relaxed, creating visible space around her neck as it appeared to elongate. As she took command of this pose she took a deep breath and when she exhaled her core engaged and her rib cage closed. Tears began to stream down her cheeks. She stood there for several minutes. She slowly opened her eyes, wiped her tears, and smiled. As her eyes met mine, I invited her to put words to that experience. She said, "I'm not sure anyone has ever seen me the way I just saw myself."

## MOVEMENT RX: ACCESSING THE VERTICAL PLANE

*Directions:*   Find a doorway to stand in.

       Place your feet in each bottom corner and reach your arms to the adjacent top corners. Allow yourself to take up space in this vertical plane. Play with the space above your head and below your knees, oscillating between the two. Continue to move until you feel your core engaging.

       Try adding breath to lubricate and support this movement exploration.

*Dosage:*   Once daily or as needed.

*Side Effects:*   Increased self-awareness with regard to identity and core beliefs.

# TAKEAWAYS

* You have to identify your place of departure before you can choose your destination.

* Looking at how you move and the nuances of your movements—in addition to which qualities you are drawn to—can take you to new heights of awareness and understanding with regard to how your movement impacts your mood and mental health.

* A greater range in movement correlates to a greater range of emotional capacity.

* Some people are flexible in their minds. Some people are flexible in their bodies. The goal is to be someone who is both.

# 6

## UNLOCKING COGNITIVE
## POTENTIAL

*The limits of our language do not
define the limits of our cognition.*
—ELLIOT W. EISNER

If chapter 4 is the heart of this book, then this chapter is the soul. Much of the work and experiences described in this chapter are the very foundation for this book's existence. For the first five years of my professional career, I focused solely on working with individuals impacted by dementia, more specifically by Alzheimer's disease. Through this work I realized very early on that movement allowed these clients to transcend many of the difficulties they faced due to cognitive decline inherent in the diagnosis. Verbal communication or difficulty communicating through language in general was an overwhelming symptom for most clients. At the root of this wasn't so much their inability to communicate, but more so the inability of people around them to understand what they were trying to communicate. Dance/movement therapy became the catalyst for bridging the communication gap and providing a platform for clients to identify, understand, and express their emotional needs.

Dance/movement therapy with older adults in general improves a person's sense of well-being and ability to cope with psychosocial stress often caused by issues of aging. It allows older adults to experience a superior sense of oneness with others, and improved self-esteem and communication.[1] Communication is made possible for many reasons, one being the atmosphere in which the dance/movement therapy occurs: a place between fantasy and reality. This imaginative place that furthers the exploration of movement is also used to increase an individual's movement repertoire. Remember that when we increase our movement repertoire or profile, we widen our window of tolerance and can improve regulation of emotions. An increased movement repertoire enables more nonverbal communication between individuals with dementia and with their caregivers.[2]

Studies have shown that dance in general supports and preserves "intellectual, emotional and motor functions" in individuals living with dementia and that communication between people with dementia was maintained through social dancing.[3] The most noteworthy finding is the emotional response that occurs when these individuals' bodies were engaged and moving. Movements facilitated "a positive physical experience" that allowed individuals "to forget their somatic impairments."[4]

Unfortunately it became more and more evident, as I worked in various memory care settings, that movement and dance specifically were not a priority. After all, the thinking went, how can we expect someone to dance if they cannot even stand or lift their head? Most nursing care facilities end up being more of a holding space for those living out the last years of their lives instead of a place where activity and life-giving interactions occur.

While that viewpoint is shifting, again movement is still focused on exercise and cardiovascular activity. Creativity in general still needs to be prioritized. Movement in all its forms, especially for those with cognitive and movement differences, is vital for expression, socialization, and communication. Movement is a way to navigate many of the cognitive symptoms, creating potential for cognition, memory, and expression.

## How I Got Here

In my graduate program for dance/movement therapy and counseling, I was placed in a yearlong internship with older adults living with memory impairment. I had some personal experience with dementia but wasn't quite sure what to expect; however, I knew right away that this was where I was meant to be. I found such ease working with older adults and appreciated the slower pace, as well as the wealth of knowledge and experience housed in their bodies, not just their minds. Throughout the years I moved with and was moved by brilliant doctors, inventors, educators, and artists, not to mention great-grandparents, mothers, husbands, and children. These lived experiences and identities were housed in their bodies and I was moved by their presence every day.

After several years working in nursing homes, senior centers, and day programs focusing on movement and dance as a means of emotional expression and an outlet for creativity, I was ready to venture into private practice. It was never a question of when, but rather how. I anticipated joining a group counseling practice, but at the time none of them placed as much importance on the body and they were more interested in traditional forms of psychotherapy. Adamant about using the title I spent years and a great deal of money earning, it occurred to me that I might very well have to create a practice myself centering around movement and dance as a therapeutic vessel for mental health.

I remembered a seminar I attended when I was a case manager at a reputable senior center in the North Shore of Chicago. The guest speaker was a social worker who worked in a neurologist's office. She met with individuals who were newly diagnosed with dementia and other cognitive disorders. I thought, "This is what I want to do!" I introduced myself to her after she spoke and asked her for some advice on how to break into this world of private practice. Years later, I decided to reach out to her, and this would change everything! She connected me to the director of the leading neurological and Alzheimer's disease center in Chicago. I remember calling this individual and asking if I could come in and speak to her team about the power of dance/movement therapy with dementia.

To my surprise she said that I could come in during lunch and speak with the small but mighty team.

We scheduled a meeting, and before I knew it, I was in the clinic with this team of social workers. I introduced myself and explained the ins and outs of dance/movement therapy. And then I asked them a simple question: "What happens when a patient you are seeing in the clinic can no longer speak or make sense verbally of what is happening or how they are feeling?" The team members looked at each other and one said, "We terminate therapy with the patient." This didn't surprise me, as we have been led to believe that once a person can no longer speak, they must have nothing to say. I simply replied, "That is when movement is necessary."

Just because someone cannot speak, doesn't mean they have nothing to say. That is often when someone has the most to say and little opportunity to say it. In fact, when individuals have difficulty communicating verbally—whether an infant, a child on the spectrum, or an adult with dementia—they must rely on nonverbal communication, on movement. This is frequently misunderstood and then misdirected. Donna Newman-Bluestein, dance/movement therapist, educator, and certified movement analyst, says, "If your attempts to communicate are misunderstood and thought to be symptomatic of dementia rather than communicative, it is likely that they'll be disregarded. And then you'll have to make your movement quicker, stronger, more direct. And those will be considered behaviors."[5] While Newman-Bluestein is referring to dementia, this applies to everyone. If we are not understood, or worse, invalidated, the body will find ways to speak up and out.

**BODY AWARE BREAK** Have you ever played charades? Next time you need to ask someone for something, try asking them using only your body; no words! How would you convey that message? Furthermore, what happens in your body when your needs are misconstrued or disregarded? How do your feelings show up in your body?

Working with my clients, I didn't see behaviors. I saw raw emotions bubbling beneath the surface like a sealed soda can that had been shaken. These individuals just wanted their needs met—to be heard, supported, and to feel safe. Movement became the catalyst for untapped potential with regard to emotional regulation, expression, and creativity. Famed dancer Mikhail Baryshnikov said, "When a body moves, it's the most revealing thing. Dance for me a minute, and I'll tell you who you are." Only I didn't have to tell them. Through movement my clients found a way back to themselves, back home to the mind through the body.

In my internship that's what we did. We danced to communicate who we were and what we needed. What began with clients in my internship eventually turned into working with private clients. I'm reminded of my first private client, a woman in her early seventies living with Alzheimer's disease. Her passion and love for God kept her going. Unfortunately, she was asked to leave her congregation for "behaviors," including boisterous singing and dancing, that were seen as disruptive and inappropriate. I met with her in her home in Bronzeville. It took many sessions for her to feel comfortable moving with me as there was paranoia, some hallucinations, and overall skepticism of my presence—which was quite understandable as I was not a familiar face or presence. I did my best to take her lead and witnessed through body cues when she needed space as well as when she was willing to engage. I'll never forget the first time she reached for my hand as we danced together in her living room. It was short but impactful. We stood across from one another as she reached out for my hand, and we moved side to side to a common rhythm. She looked at me and smiled as she sang to the music and embodied the words of Aretha Franklin's "Natural Woman."

Every week her living room became the church. We moved to familiar hymns, which eventually evolved into Motown and James Brown (her favorite singer) medleys. She came alive, and when it came time to sit and catch our breath, she would tell me all about God. He was her best friend. This went on for many years until her passing. It wasn't always easy for her, or me for that matter. She had good days and bad days. Her family struggled as so many caregivers and families do, but movement gave her a quality of life. It provided access to meaning and purpose. I will never forget her. I can still to this day recall her movements and mannerisms as we danced together. She said to me one day, "I don't worry. I pray." I keep her words with me always—words that others thought to be inaccessible through traditional methods become possible through movement. Words that might not have been heard otherwise give me comfort and peace.

Potential for connection to self, other, and our environment is always possible. Movement is the way to access it. This chapter may be inspired by older adults, but the benefits of movement for unlocking cognitive potential apply to all ages and abilities. Potential belongs to everyone.

## Potential Defined

Potential is defined as "having or showing the capacity to become or develop into something in the future." The future can be twenty years from now or twenty seconds from now. Whether someone is five years old or ninety-five years old, potential is accessible. There is potential in a lifetime, but also in a weekly therapy session. As long as there is space to create, there is potential. It seems to me that we confuse time and age for potential. While more time can support more room for potential, it is not needed. Nowhere in the above definition does it imply age with regard to potential. Everyone deserves the opportunity to access the capacity of becoming or doing something in the future.

Obviously, physical abilities and capabilities change due to natural aging or a life event, but that does not dictate potential. If movement is a catalyst for change, then it can also support adaptation during life's greatest challenges. Consider not only the potential to become something, but also individual potential for expression, creativity, emotional regulation, and cognition. Again, movement can support agency, motivation, and purpose by connecting to our embodied experiences and sensations.

Cognition is the mental process of gaining knowledge through thought, experience, or the senses. Let me clarify that this is any knowledge and does not only pertain to neurotypical development. Cognitive potential is the possibility of gaining that knowledge. There are many factors that influence one's potential for understanding or acquiring knowledge. Attention, focus, and awareness are vital, especially when creating and retaining memories. If we are not present and aware, memory is impacted. There's a reason that students perform better when movement and even dance are introduced into the curriculum. Research shows that movement influences cognition. Just ten minutes of walking a day can improve memory retention and overall academic performance.[6] Remember that how we move impacts the experiences we have, therefore when we invite in more movement, we invite in the potential for more experiences. More experiences provide more opportunity for new thoughts and acquisition of knowledge for cognitive potential.

To take a body aware approach when it comes to cognitive potential means embracing an embodied framework: embodied cognition. Embodied cognition for purposes of this book refers to the notion that your thoughts don't just live in your mind, but throughout your body. Cognitive potential is accessible for everyone with a body. Regardless of developmental or cognitive abilities, it is vital that we begin to shift how we embrace and engage with movement in order to support potential—potential to learn, connect, communicate, and express.

Cognitive potential is limited by disembodied knowledge, but it's infinite when we involve the body. It would be like learning to read English if you were only given thirteen letters. It might be possible, but there would be a lot missing. Embodiment, actively being in your body, provides access to the whole alphabet. Not only can you read, but you can create new vocabulary. We can forever develop cognitive potential by challenging our bodies to move in new ways.

The beautiful part is again that there is no right way, but rather creating opportunity based on individual needs and abilities. We've already explored how changing our definition of movement helps reframe what it can look like with regard to mental health. Let's explore why movement works with regard to tapping into and unlocking potential.

## How Movement Supports Cognitive Potential

The right brain develops first in utero, and it supports nonverbal communication between mother and child.[7] This I believe is the reason why movement is the key that unlocks cognitive potential. By using movement we access the right brain, which taps into the primitive modes of communication—the areas of the brain that are accessible even through something like a dementia diagnosis. Once we have activated the right brain, we can encourage connection to the left brain through movement that supports communication across the corpus callosum, a thick bundle of nerve fibers that connect the two hemispheres. Crossing the midline of the body through gentle touch, a hug, or tapping facilitates crossing this midline of the brain. We can literally encourage left brain function by connecting to the right brain first.

I believe there is evidence that just as the development of movement patterns supports cognitive development, when brain development is stunted or deteriorates, so do these movement patterns. For example, I hypothesized during my graduate program internship that as Alzheimer's disease progressed, the developmental movement patterns in each individual regressed as well and that if we could reintroduce these patterns, we could enhance cognitive potential—at least in the moment. For those who may not be familiar, Alzheimer's disease literally leads to deterioration of the brain, creating holes where matter and activity used to reside. Essentially, as the brain continues to lose its connectivity, this is mirrored in the loss of connectivity in the body.

I witnessed this in how my clients would march or even walk. Remember from chapter 4 that Cross-Lateral Connectivity, seen in walking or marching, is "the most complex pattern in the basic developmental sequence."[8] This is evolutionarily the most advanced body pattern, since it requires the integration of all previous patterns. Physically, as one arm swings, the opposite leg engages and vice versa. What I noticed in the participants was homologous marching. As one arm would swing, the same leg would engage. (Try it. It's not easy to do, especially if you are used to cross-lateral movement.) Referring back to chapter 4, this is known as

Body-Half Connectivity, where "one half of the body learns to stabilize so that the other can become more mobile."[9] I saw this reflected not only in the body movements of my clients, but also in their thought patterns. In an individual who has access to cross-lateral movement, thought patterns are more integrated and advanced. Someone can recognize opposing ideas, see both sides, and draw their own conclusions. With my clients their thought patterns were more binary, meaning they were back to identifying a side: right-wrong, left-right, etc. Their thought patterns, like their movements, were dis-integrated. Their understanding of topics and discussion were very basic, and there was little inference or exploration. This is not true for all individuals with dementia, but merely an observation that illustrates not only a correlation between how we move and how we think, but that when our movement patterns regress, so do our thought patterns.

Why is this important? I believe that encouraging participants to engage in advanced movement patterns supports their cognitive potential. I have witnessed a client go from one-word answers and remarks to full sentences with inflection and wonderment after I encouraged them to activate advanced movement patterns. Inviting an individual to touch their knee using the opposite arm and engaging in a self-hug are simple ways to encourage this advanced movement pattern. While research is needed to support this hypothesis, it is something I continue to see over and over again.

I am aware of the sweeping generalizations being made. Not all individuals living with dementia are the same, even moment to moment an individual's demeanor and behavior can change. The disease progression as well as the parts of the brain affected will vary. What is the same across the board is the stigma these individuals face as well as the idea that identity is lost and that this disease takes all dignity away from them. When we address, honor, and witness a person's movement and nonverbal communication, we acknowledge their very existence—their identity and their capacity to be, to do, and to achieve.

I once had a mentee ask me, "What is it like to work with terminal patients?" I was taken aback. I had never thought about dementia as a terminal illness. While most dementias are progressive, I myself hadn't seen it as terminal—perhaps because many of my clients on some level weren't aware of their diagnosis and lived ten or more years with it as well. They knew that something felt "off" but it wasn't always a topic of conversation. That is to say I believe that coming into my groups every day, not focusing on the limitations of the participants and the diagnosis, created room for possibility. Possibility breeds potential. Movement gives potential a seat at the table and opportunity to enhance individual expression and communication. A body aware approach encourages harnessing this power to tap into our greatest potential by embracing all the ways we move.

## Harnessing Your Cognitive Potential

No matter your cognitive abilities, movement can unlock potential. As the previous section points out, anyone—even those losing brain function—has potential. The following are suggestions that anyone can adopt to increase cognitive potential through movement. This is not to be confused with cognitive reserve, which will be discussed further in chapter 8. Movement, while accessible and possible for everyone, comes more naturally to some than others. Sometimes we need assistance and encouragement to get the ball rolling. Whether you are looking to boost performance on a job, tap into your sense of purpose, manage symptoms, or connect to your community, here are some ways to tap into your potential.

FIND YOUR RHYTHM.    Maya Angelou said, "Everything in the universe has a rhythm, everything dances." Whether it is tapping into your own inherent rhythms like the cadence of your breath or the beat of your heart or using music to explore an external rhythm, all are great jumping-off points. A syncopated rhythm especially can be a good way to engage the body. Dr. Maria Witek, Senior Birmingham Fellow in Birmingham University's Department of Music, proposes in her research that "syncopations, because they fall off the beat rather than on the beat, you can think of them as kind of opening up spaces in the rhythmic surface. And these open spaces in rhythm invite the body to fill them in through synchronized body movement."[10] Child psychiatrist Dr. Stanley Greenspan found that rhythm and timing are key components to learning and in fact have been shown to provide a foundation for emotional development. There is so much research on music for mental and emotional health. Additionally I encourage you to look into the professional field of music therapy. While the above information is in no way representative of that field, just like movement, music is another universal language that fosters connection, enhances communication, and facilitates emotional regulation.

**EXPLORE ALL MOVEMENT POSSIBLE.** When we are in pain or have limitations in our movement, we tend to fixate on them or let them dictate what we can and cannot do. It is vital that we refocus on movement that is possible in the moment. Allow your potential to flourish by embracing all the possibilities. I had a participant in one of my groups who had suffered a stroke that rendered his left side paralyzed. I remember that the first time he came to this group, a staff member made sure to tell me that he could not move his left side. Would you believe me if I told you that in the middle of the group that same client grabbed his left arm with his right hand and proceeded to lift both arms over his head? Had I discouraged him from using his left side or reinforced his limitations, the potential for movement, and therefore cognition, would have been stifled. Instead I created the opportunity for him to realize his own potential. This led to an insightful conversation and a greater sense of empowerment and self-esteem as exhibited by the client's change in posture and affect at the end of the group. Rather than fixating on the "impossible," it is imperative that we create space and opportunity to shift into "I'm possible."

**MOVE IN COMMUNITY.** You do not have to do this alone. In fact, moving with others can make moving easier and supportive. Indigenous cultures and tribes have been using the power of communal movement for thousands of years. One example is the round dance performed by the Cree peoples, which focuses on the circle as a place where people and ancestors meet, providing communal support and love.[11] The haka, a ceremonial dance in Māori culture, is performed by a group and entails "vigorous movements and stamping of the feet with rhythmically shouted accompaniment"[12] designed to show pride, strength, and unity.[13] Marian Chace, often referred to as the "Grande Dame of Dance Therapy," has incorporated group-based circular and rhythmic movement into her work. Protégés of Chace, Sharon Chaiklin and Claire Schmais, classified this as rhythmic activity, also referred to as a group rhythmic movement relationship.[14]

The contagious aspect of rhythm could mobilize even severely withdrawn patients, with safe and simple rhythmic sequences providing a medium for the externalization of otherwise chaotic and confusing emotions ... the group rhythmic movement relationship provides a structure in which thoughts and feelings are shaped, organized and released with the secure confines of both the rhythmic action (which provides repetition and mastery) and the group structure and support.[15]

**IF AT FIRST YOU DON'T SUCCEED...** The capacity for movement is always there; however, the longer you have not used it, the more time it takes to reengage those parts. You cannot expect anyone, including yourself, to jump into a movement practice or dance and "perform" at 100 percent. Not only is that dangerous but it also places judgment on how it should be done and what it should look like. We must build up to it. Remember, in order to move forward we must recognize where we are at the start—meeting ourselves in the MOveMENT. It deserves to be repeated that practice makes habit. Continue finding ways to prioritize movement in your life and your potential will unfold.

While these are just a few ways in which you can use movement to harness your own potential, like many you may suffer from a lack of motivation to get moving. Movement and motivation go hand in hand.

## Movement and Motivation

A large piece of unlocking your potential is finding the motivation to do it. Gbenaga Adebambo, author and youth advocate, says, "Movement creates momentum, momentum creates motivation."[16] Even the most successful people aren't always motivated, but they keep moving. I experienced this, as dancing through difficult times kept me moving, and while not everyone may feel called to dance, we can all move in our own ways to tap into our motivation. Furthermore we can use movement to create momentum, which helps us tap into feeling motivated. Motivation to do or be something opens avenues to potential.

Newman-Bluestein believes that "many people with dementia are unable to access motivation. They need someone, preferably everyone, to provide sufficient sensory stimulation that is culturally and personally relevant to help them to connect to their intrinsic motivation."[17] This is good news for those of us who are not diagnosed with a memory or cognitive impairment. Connecting to the present moment through sensory stimulation and movement allows us to harness our personal sense of motivation.

In this day and age of instant gratification, waiting for results isn't easy. When we see and feel change happen in real time, we are more motivated to continue. The slightest change in our movement can have large impacts on our mood, thoughts, and life overall. In fact, you may find that changes happen in the most unsuspecting places.

While conducting a study with a student from Northwestern University on the effects of dance therapy on Parkinson's disease, I was introduced to a woman who did not identify herself as a dancer. She was recommended by her neurologist to participate in the study. She was newly diagnosed and had difficulty with balance and gait in addition to fatigue. At the conclusion of the study, the participant noticed positive changes not only in all of the above symptoms but also specifically in one that surprised her: her dexterity had improved. Working on connectivities in the body fosters connection in the brain. This participant's improvement in coordination and sense of control with regard to micromovements like holding a pen, were noticeable and motivated her to continue with dance therapy after the study ended.

Moving in creative, expressive, and at times improvisational ways has the power to impact all areas of our lives. So what movement supports the creation of momentum and motivates our minds and bodies? While there is no one right answer, here's a good place to start.

BREATH. Let's start with the involuntary movement that is happening right now as you read this. Acknowledging, identifying, and increasing the awareness of your breathing is the foundation for expanding your movement potential. Dr. Jamie Marich, creator of Dancing Mindfulness, says that "we can give breath to new connections, to new ideas. All innovation and creation is born of breath."[18] This is a poignant display of how tuning into breath allows us to tap into the momentum needed to create.

ENGAGE YOUR SENSES. As mentioned by Newman-Bluestein, sensory stimulation can signal motivation. Not only does engaging the senses connect us to the present moment but it also sparks cerebral activity. During playtime, combining the senses supports the development of cognitive skills. Young children store memories through sensory experiences, which in turn help them gain knowledge and understanding.[19] Smelling smoke can alert us to danger, which can motivate us to move toward safety. Not feeling like getting up or "moving," so to speak? Tune into what you hear, taste, smell, see, and feel. That alone can spark movement that will result in physical momentum.

TAP INTO YOUR PERSONAL RHYTHM. Notice whatever rhythm already exists in your body. The beat of your heart, the rise and fall of your breath, even the blink of an eye is all you need to get moving. Allow these inherent rhythms to "move" you to a new position.

ACCESS PLANES OF MOVEMENT TO CONNECT TO MOMENTUM. We can create momentum by moving in certain directions. Revisit the previous chapter to breathe or stretch into different dimensions. You might notice that a certain direction is connected to your intrinsic motivation.

GIVE YOURSELF PERMISSION TO RESIST AND REST. Resisting the urge to go, do, and be can ironically pave the way for momentum.

Rest is needed, and for so many it is a last thought. Motivation doesn't come from one kind of movement. It comes from any movement, and that movement can even be the still, quiet posture or gesture of rest and relaxation. Motivation is often associated with productivity. I came across an article entitled "Rest as Resistance: A Guidebook to 24/7 Capitalism." Author Billie Walker states that "the exhaustion of society is created by the pressure to be constantly productive: the need to be busy. . . . Rest is integral to your own political and creative freedom."[20] Creative freedom is exactly what you need to access your potential. When we rest we create space for thought and ideas, which can lead to innovation. Ironically when we slow down we can actually enhance our productivity and focus. There is power in being, not just doing.

Movement is magical, and its power is within everyone. Movement can instill agency, support resilience, and empower you to own your movement qualities as your superpowers. We've redefined movement and uncovered how to expand our own affinities to movement. Now we will explore how those combined facilitate new perspectives, support diversity, and pave the way for transformation.

## Unlocking Cognitive Potential in Motion

Eleanor, a ninety-four-year-old client, displayed typical symptoms of Alzheimer's disease. She had severe memory impairment, was not oriented to time or place, and repeatedly checked her purse for her ID. On this particular day, Eleanor was in a group consisting of seven women. After a brief body warm-up, which included a check-in of each body part, the group was invited to pretend that the space in front of them was a blank canvas and their arms were the paintbrushes. I played soft classical music in the background.

Eleanor, a classically trained pianist and very artistic and creative woman, was enthralled in the painting process. I could see the wheels in her head turning as she painted the air in front of her. After the movement portion came to a close, the group began processing what had taken place. I asked what people had painted, and Eleanor proceeded to explain this beautiful scene in her mind. Eleanor had painted a boat for the group to go on a cruise. She was then asked what her favorite part about that cruise was, and she said, "The fresh air and the reflection in the water." The group was invited to feel "the fresh air." Many members closed their eyes and took a slow deep breath. When asked what she saw in the water, Eleanor replied that she saw a reflection of herself at twenty-five with her man's arms around her waist. As she explained this, tears began to form in her eyes and she hesitated for a moment. Eleanor concluded that she felt good about the memories, even though they brought tears to her eyes. The group concluded and moments later Eleanor opened her purse and resumed looking for her ID.

## MOVEMENT RX: MOVING FOR POTENTIAL

*Directions:* Let me introduce you to something I learned in graduate school called WOMMPing (W-water, O-oxygen, M-marching, M-midline, P-pretzel). This experience was developed by Marcia Parsons, a dance/movement therapist and professor emeritus at University of Wisconsin-Milwaukee. This is designed to move your body in a way that sparks connection in your brain to enhance focus, support attention, and reenergize mind and body.

Step 1: Begin by drinking water.

Step 2: Take three deep belly breaths.

Step 3: Begin marching in place using the same arm and same leg (*homolateral*).

Step 4: After marching homolaterally, shift to marching with your opposite arm and opposite leg (*cross-lateral*).

Step 5: Rotate palms inward, cross arms, and clasp hands. Pull arms toward chest and through (if possible). Simultaneously cross your legs while standing (if possible). Be sure to try crossing arms and legs the other way as well. This might be similar to Eagle Pose in yoga.

*Dosage:*    For use as needed.

*Side Effects:*    Greater awareness, focus, and attention. May increase confidence and productivity.

## TAKEAWAYS

* Just because someone cannot speak doesn't mean they have nothing to say.
* As long as there is space to create, there is potential.
* Remember that how we move impacts the experiences we have; therefore, when we invite in more movement we invite in the potential for more experiences.
* No matter your cognitive abilities, movement can unlock potential.
* The slightest change in our movement can have large impacts on our mood, thoughts, and life overall.

# Part 3

# TRANSFORMATION THROUGH MOVEMENT

# 7

# PERSPECTION

*We don't see things as they are, we see them as we are.*

—ANAÏS NIN, French-Cuban-American diarist

We have looked at how you move and how adaptations to your movement facilitate behavioral changes. Now it's time to put the pieces together. Integrating what you've learned from parts 1 and 2 into your life can lead to transformation. Transformation seems like a fancy word for change, but when I focus on the word and notice where it elicits a response in my body, I notice a distinct difference. Change feels to be more in the moment, moving from one thing to the next, and may be temporary or fleeting. Transformation feels deeper. In my body, it is slower, stronger, and more direct. Transformation is embodied change. It is conscious, intentional, and everlasting. When I look to transform something there is a realization that it will be forever changed. In his book, *Managing Transitions: Making the Most of Change,* Dr. William Bridges writes, "Change is situational. Transition is psychological."[1] I believe transformation is both. To be truly transformed one must engage the mind and body.

That is what part 3 is about: transformation. We will examine how movement alters our perception, enhances resilience, and has the capacity to support our unique abilities and differences. Part 3 ends with a chapter dedicated to helping you put it all into practice where you can not only gain more insight as well as daily practices but also you can find ways to translate this material into real-life scenarios.

Let's look at your potential transformation from before picking up this book to the end and beyond. You may have been living in avoidance—avoiding emotions, responsibility, relationships, people, mirrors, etc. If this book teaches you anything, let it be this: you can go from avoidance to abundance by embracing the healing properties of *dance*. Remember that from a body aware perspective, dance isn't a specific technique, skill, or stylized choreography. As Anna Halprin, cofounder of the Tamalpa Insitute, an internationally recognized nonprofit organization that offers expressive arts training programs and workshops, said, "Movement reaches our deepest nature, and dance creatively expresses it."[2] Dance is movement and movement is life, therefore, dance is life! By embracing movement and *all* movement that is possible in your body at any given moment, you have the ability to go from a place of avoi*dance* to a place of abun*dance*.

Keep in mind that this too is a practice. The goal is to make abundance more accessible, not to eliminate avoidance altogether. It is important to acknowledge the avoidance and challenge how it keeps us small. Owning our ingrained habits and intentionally creating opportunities for new outlooks is how we foster transformation. Ultimately you will experience a shift in perspective facilitated by consistently listening to and referencing your body's language. This is what I call *perspection*.

> **BODY AWARE BREAK** What does avoidance look and feel like? Take a few minutes to try it on in your body. Now try the same thing with abundance.
>
> What differences do you notice between the two in your body? Where do they exist in your body?

*Perspection* is a new word I happened upon in a supervision session with a dance/movement therapy intern. The words *perspective* and *introspection* seemed to morph in my mind and came out of my mouth as perspection. I chuckled, but actually sat with it for a moment and felt like I had stumbled onto something that I have continued to share with my clients. It is a work in progress, but something I feel necessary to share as it is inherent to a body aware practice.

Perspection is defined as a shift in perspective facilitated by a new awareness derived from the body. Essentially it is a new outlook resulting from changes that take place as a result of being body aware. As I have continued to sit with this term I have come to realize that perspection combines four elements: perspective, perception, interoception, and introspection.

## Perspective and Perception

*Perspective* is the way you see or understand something, while *perception* is the ability to see, hear, or become aware of something. Both traditionally correspond to cognitive awareness, but here, we're going to focus on how we can cultivate perspective through the body in a way that changes our perception. First let's look at how we can change perspective through the body. You can become more aware of your current perspective by noticing the sounds, smells, and sights around you.

When encouraging clients to explore perspective, this is my "go-to" intervention: I invite the client to move to another place in the therapy room. I then invite them to take notice through their senses of their new surroundings. We can talk about what is different, similar, comfortable, uncomfortable, etc. But the most important thing I believe is allowing the body to shift in order to see that other perspectives are possible, and more important, perspective doesn't change unless we invite in new experiences. And remember from chapter 4 that experiences start with movement. When we move in new and different ways, we allow the opportunity to recognize different perspectives.

I was working with a young woman who was struggling to get back on her feet, literally and figuratively, after a serious car accident. While meeting outdoors during the pandemic in 2020, I invited her to approach a large tree. As she stepped right up against the tree's large trunk, I asked her to comment on what she saw. She saw what was right in front of her: the tree. I then asked her to take a few steps back and reflect on what she could see now. She began to engage her neck and eyes as she scanned the area, looking up into the tree branches, down at the roots, and around at the surrounding plants. Her eyes widened as she let out a great sigh. The exercise, she said, showed her that the tree reminded her of her accident, of the point in time that changed everything. Focusing on it so closely was preventing her from seeing what was around her. But stepping back to take a different view never seemed like an option because in order to move on she assumed she needed to move forward. Trouble was she couldn't move forward with an obstacle in her direct path. It was only after she stepped back that she began to walk around the tree and find a path to her future.

When we invite in new perspectives through the body, we expand our perception in the mind. Additionally, being able to see other points of view allows us to empathize and understand others' situations. When you have a sense of how something feels in your body, you can own your personal experience and acknowledge that not every body feels the exact same way. For example, we all have the capacity to feel anger, but where we feel it and how it manifests may vary from person to person. I may feel it in my chest as a burning sensation, while someone else may feel it as heat or tension in their arms and hands. When we try on others' emotions, meaning put them into our bodies and viscerally experience them from their physical frame of reference, it changes us. This is how empathy is created—by walking or moving in another person's metaphorical shoes, also known as their body. You can create space for understanding instead of judgment by being present to internal sensations in your own body as a response to others' in theirs.

Let me offer an example. While working with a client, the subject of rage came up in many sessions. It was actually a quite prevalent reaction identified by the client. I recognized that my own perception of rage was different from what they perceived as rage. I invited the client to display or show me in their body through a posture, gesture, or sequence of movements what rage felt like to them. With the client's permission I mirrored this display as closely as possible in order to preserve the integrity of their experience. This allowed me to feel what it was like to the client as well as provide an opportunity for the client to see how the rage was externalized or represented in their body. Bringing their sensing of rage into my body helped me see the client's perspective as well as validate their experience.

Sensations, such as "feeling cold" or "feeling hungry," are literally perceptions that result from something happening to the body. Perception relies on our senses as it is the process of becoming aware or understanding something through our senses. For example, the smell of smoke can be perceived as danger of a fire. Perception can also be a way of interpreting something. The way we see and interpret things is dependent on our location, position, and understanding or misunderstanding of the world around us. We can change the way we understand and interpret our world by looking at how we move through it. Change the way you move and the way you perceive things changes as well. Furthermore, when we move we engage our senses, ultimately facilitating a change in perception.

## Interoception

Interoception for the purpose of this book is defined as the perception of sensations from inside the body. Examples include a growling stomach, a full bladder, and tense muscles. While this term has gained popularity in the last twenty years, its first known usage in publication appears in Charles Scott Sherrington's book *The Integrative Action of the Nervous System* in 1906.[3] Regardless, you do not need a formal definition to grasp this sense. Anytime you pay attention to an internal sensation, you are tapping into your interoceptive sense.

When I sat down to write this section, I suddenly felt stuck with regard to defining this sense; and when I took time to reflect, I realized that this section, while important, is the newest to me. Like you, I have access to this sense whether I'm conscious of it or not, but I don't personally have a long history of being aware of it. In fact like many of you, I resisted and denied many of the sensations in my body.

Being body aware has allowed me to hone my interoceptive capabilities. The more I embraced the paradigm that my body holds all experiences, the more willing and able I was—and am—to acknowledge and make time to be with the sensations inside. This is what I referred to in chapter 3 as your body's language. I believe three constructs need to be present in order to intentionally explore interoception: safety, curiosity, and self-compassion.

We need to feel safe in order to explore the unknown, the uncertain, and the uncomfortable. At the very least we need to have access to resources that allow us to find a sense of safety in our bodies. When we have a safe space to come home to, we are more able to venture out and explore uncharted emotional territory. While we cannot always control our environment, we can look for elements that contribute to security, stability, and support. When we have a sense of how those feel internally, we can decipher when they are present externally, and if they're not, then we can proactively take steps to ensure our own safety. This can be removing ourselves from a particular environment, setting and holding boundaries, or reaching out for support from a trusted confidant. Safety is vital for surviving, but internal safety is vital for thriving. In order to trust our intuition, our environment, and the people in it, we must tap into our safety. Dr. Amber Gray, creator of Polyvagal-informed dance/movement therapy, says, "Trust is built on safety, and relationships are built on trust. Safety begins in the body."[4] This would be a good time to revisit Gray's interventions in chapter 4.

They say curiosity killed the cat. This implies that inquisitiveness leads to danger or harm. But I believe it is vital to be curious about our behaviors if we want to be the best version of ourselves. This is why safety is needed, because it provides a foundation for discerning when danger is in fact present; otherwise, we can go our whole lives stifling our curiosity. Becoming curious about why we move and act the way we do allows us to challenge those ingrained habits and to ultimately create lasting change.

Self-compassion is needed in order to relinquish the criticism and judgment that keeps us from making mistakes and embracing change. We will undoubtedly fall into old habits as we seek to embrace new ones.

It is the ability to limit the judgment and find compassion through the learning process that creates a path to transformation. Compassion can be harnessed during moments of reflection and introspection.

Dance/movement therapist Fatina Hindi states, "Researchers are finding evidence that supports the hypothesis that one's ability to attend to interoceptive sensation is correlative to one's ability to experience a range of emotions and feel efficacy in navigating those emotions."[5] When we have a greater understanding of our own embodied feelings, we have a greater ability to express and manage them. This will be explored more in chapter 8 and is the basis for what I believe is resilience through the body.

## Introspection

Introspection is the examination or observation of one's own mental and emotional processes. This is something I have a lot of experience with. I always associated it with being an only child, alone with my thoughts a lot. Growing up I wasn't always curious about why I did what I did, but I was very aware of the voices telling me how to feel about what I did. You may be familiar with those voices. They are the echoes from your upbringing: the caregivers, authority figures, and educators who become our internal monologue. This was the only sense I operated from for a long time. Always overanalyzing, overthinking, and at times obsessing over thoughts and actions in what I now know was an attempt to control the uncontrollable.

While introspection is usually associated with mindfulness, there is great opportunity to use the body to observe emotional processes. For example, rather than only asking "what is on your mind?" consider asking "what is on your body?" This creates space and intention for introspection with a focus on where in the body these emotions may be held. So what might this look like? Notice for a moment what emotional load your body is currently carrying. Are you under any stress? If so, notice where that shows up in your body. It may be through a tight jaw, tension in your chest or shoulders, maybe even a lack of movement in your torso. Perhaps you are feeling fatigued or overwhelmed. How are these feelings differentiated in the body? In other words, without relying on your mind to decipher what you are feeling, notice what is happening on a body level that suggests you are feeling that way.

If you are not exactly sure of what you are feeling with regard to an emotion, you can begin by noticing sensations in the body. Identifying these sensations can allow you to understand what you are feeling. With the anger example previously mentioned, perhaps you aren't aware you are angry. You feel heat in your hands, and the more you allow yourself to notice "what is on your body," the more you are able to decipher what emotion is connected to that particular sensation in that particular moment. Asking "what is on your body" enables you to connect a visceral experience with an emotion. Keep in mind that different emotions may experience similar sensations. I feel a fluttering in my chest when I am excited, but also when I'm anxious. This is why it is important to include perception and perspective, paying attention to the context and environment.

Introspection is a good place to start when creating awareness with regard to our emotions and thoughts. For those of you who, like me, may spend much time in your headspace, introspection can pave the way for interoception.

## Implications of Perspection

There are many benefits to increasing one's perspection. Perspection paves the way for more resilience, empathy, and connection. This doesn't just translate to the individual but to a person's networks, community, and habitat.

You may be familiar with the saying "be the change you want to see." I say, "Embody the change you want to see": breathe, move, and express the energy and actions you wish to see in the world and in others. After all, how can we expect the world to be in balance when the people inhabiting it are not?

### Implication #1: Healthier Environment

So often we are a product of our environment. If we are raised in a chaotic atmosphere then that becomes the norm, reinforcing that our external environment generates our internal homeostasis. What if your internal landscape could influence the external environment? News flash; it does!

The idea that we are deeply connected with nature is not a novel concept. North American Indigenous peoples and First Nations have modeled the importance of connection, communication, and collaboration with nature and the universe for thousands of years. Chief Seattle, a Suquamish and Duwamish chief, was quoted to have said, "Humankind has not woven the web of life. We are but one thread within it. Whatever we do to the web, we do to ourselves. All things are bound together. All things connect." I would add that the opposite is also true: whatever we do to ourselves, we do to the web.

Another example is that of the culture of Australia's Aboriginal and Torres Strait Islanders (ATSI) who lived in harmony with nature for over forty thousand years before being invaded. ATSI people do not view land as something to be owned. On the contrary, they view the "land as owning them."[6] They live with the land as if with a mother figure, and focus on preservation, as her health is directly related to protection.[7]

Preservation is significant in Hinduism as well. In Hinduism man is forbidden from harming the land. In fact Sanskrit mantras are recited by millions of Hindus daily to show esteem for natural elements inherent to the land. Tree-hugging, initially identified as the Chipko movement, started in India and was molded by the Hindu faith.[8]

There is an emerging field in Western therapeutic practice called eco-somatics that melds embodiment practices with ecological consciousness. While *soma,* taken from Ancient Greek, translates to "body," adding *eco-* starts the dialogue of incorporating "an organism's relationship to its environment." According to dance and somatic educator Susan Bauer, author of "Body and Earth as One," "truly ecosomatic approaches intentionally ground our practices in the body by encouraging direct sensory perception of one's body as the natural environment."[9, 10, 11]

It is no coincidence that humans and the Earth contain the same amount of water, approximately 70 percent of our bodies.[12] This so beautifully illustrates the connection addressed by Chief Seattle. If the elements inside of us, the ones also found in the Earth, are out of alignment, then the Earth will be as well. Katie Asmus, founder of the Somatic Wilderness Therapy Institute, says, "What we do impacts the planet and the planet's health impacts us."[13] Essentially, how we move impacts the planet. When we move with more intention and attention, we are more conscientious of what influences our movements and how our movements impact the world around us.

As the above examples show, fostering perspective not only creates opportunity for a healthier planet, but a healthier internal environment as well. Having a healthy relationship with the internal sensations of our body allows us to address emotional concerns faster as they are present in the body before they enter the mind. When we are aware we can address and manage our feelings faster. Additionally, with increased awareness it takes us less time to recover. Something that once may have occupied my mind and body for two weeks now takes forty-eight hours to unpack and process. This is one thing that supports resilience, a theme that will be discussed in the next chapter.

> **BODY AWARE BREAK** Take a moment to find stability in your body. This could be sitting down, leaning against a sturdy wall, or standing on your own two feet. Notice what is needed externally for you to feel stable. Now find a way to safely explore instability. This could be raising your heels off the floor, leaning or bending over, or playing with your center of gravity. What do you notice about your environment when you feel unstable?

## Implication #2: Healthier Relationships

The ability to be more aware of our bodies as well as our emotions and feelings impacts not only ourselves, but also the people we interact with. As mentioned previously, we are able to set limits, show up for others, and take responsibility for what emotionally is ours and what is not. Think about the relationship you have with your body. Do you have open communication with it? Do you listen to it, ignore it, silence it? Are you aware of the signals it is giving off to you or to the people around you? Now consider your relationships. Are there any similarities between how you communicate with your body and how you communicate with the people in your life? Perhaps you have never looked at it in this light. We are all familiar with the Golden Rule, "treat others as you would want to be treated." The same applies to how you treat the relationship you have with your body. You have to treat your body the way you want others to treat it.

You see, when our perspective changes, so does the way we interact with people. Author of *The Body Is Not an Apology,* Sonya Renee Taylor says, "It is through our own transformed relationship with our bodies that we become champions for other bodies on this planet."[14] When we accept and love ourselves, as Taylor puts it, "radically," we can learn to accept and love others, and they can do the same for us in return. Additionally we can care better for others because we are taking care of ourselves. Perspection leads to greater self-care, which has the ability to shed light on our own value, worthiness, and self-respect.

## Implication #3: Improved Patient Care/Advocacy

When we have a better understanding of who we are, we can advocate for our needs. Perspection even translates to the medical community. With more emphasis on perspection, physicians and wellness practitioners would have more empathy for patients as well as the ability to implement their own self-care. In her thesis entitled *Examining the Connection between Spirituality and Embodiment in Medical Education,* dance/movement therapist Katie Bellamy concluded that with experiential learning and the implementation of embodiment techniques, medical students were provided the opportunity to decrease reliance on cognitive approaches and increase mind-body awareness, ultimately paving the way for empathy.[15]

I remember speaking to a group of medical students at a health and wellness conference in Chicago. Following experiential hands-on practices, students began to see how their own body awareness contributed to their bedside manner and burnout. Imagine how health care would change if our physicians and the medical community emphasized the importance of communication and connection to the body. I will never forget the first encounter I had with my current primary care physician. I had many years of struggling to find a doctor who really listened to me and didn't just say what they read in a recent article or prescribe the latest medication brought in by a pharmaceutical rep. She began with the typical inquiries: family history, activity level, recreational activity, etc. She asked me, "Do you smoke?" I responded no. "Do you drink?" No. Then she followed it with, "Are you religious or spiritual?" I assumed that was a follow-up from why I don't drink, so I said, "Well, I am religious, but that's not why I don't drink." She chuckled and explained that she was interested in my spiritual life because that is a part of health. I about fainted! In all my thirty years up to that point, I had never had a doctor ask me that question. I felt my body relax and release all of this tension, anxiety, and confusion from years of being doubted and made to feel as if someone knew more about my body that I did.

Empathy within the medical community often occurs when a physician or medical student has had a personal experience that allows them to know how it feels to be in the patient's circumstance. Research suggests that while medical students may have a greater propensity toward empathy, their ability to empathize declines as the demands for academic knowledge increase. This can be an attempt to manage or mismanage the anxiety, stress, and workload, but also speaks to the lack of focus and education in Western medicine with regard to empathy.[16] Prioritizing mental and emotional well-being for medical professionals is necessary to provide holistic care. Teaching the medical community to reference their own body knowledge and wisdom empowers them to empower their patients to do the same.

Perspection creates a ripple effect. Much like a virus can spread from person to person, so too can kindness and empathy created from honing perspection. By taking a look at how we embody or physically deny our own compassion, care, and dignity, we create opportunities to model it for others.

How different might the world look if everyone practiced a body aware approach? Changing not only how you see something but how you feel something in your skin, muscles, and organs is a concept lost on so many these days. Our bodies are not simply instruments of physical strength, endurance, or aesthetics. Our bodies hold infinite wisdom, and when resourced, can provide new perspectives and understanding, opening us up to the world and its challenges. Through the body and mind we can overcome adversity and embrace resilience.

## Perspection in Motion

Rachelle came into the session in a hurried manner. She began walking quickly around the room as she spoke rapidly, firing off the events of the day and week. I invited her to notice her pace, timing, and rhythm. Still moving rather quickly, she began to call out what she noticed. "I am pacing. I'm moving fast. I can't slow down." I asked her what would happen if she slowed down. She replied, "I'll lose control." I replied, "What would it look like to lose control?" Rachelle began to walk faster, swinging her arms, shaking her hands frantically, until she stopped in her tracks. She froze for about fifteen seconds, short of breath and bound in her upper body. Then slowly her shoulders relaxed, her chin lifted, and her knees softened. She stood for a minute as she closed her eyes and took a deep breath. When her eyes opened, I invited her to speak to what she just experienced. She mentioned that she always thought that if she kept moving she could control how much or how little she felt. "I thought stopping altogether would feel out of control, that all the emotions would come flooding in. But in my attempt to gain control, I noticed I am actually out of control. When I slow down, I connect to my power, strength, and myself. When I slow down I am in control."

**MOVEMENT RX: NEW PERSPECTIVES**

*Directions:*    Find a comfortable place in the room. You can sit or stand. Soften your gaze for a moment and focus on your breath. Draw your attention to your head and allow your head to be the part of your body that initiates or leads your movement. Replicate this with your chest, hips, and any other parts of your body that pique your interest. What do you notice internally when you allow different parts of your body to lead your movement?

*Dosage:*    Once or twice a week or as needed.

*Side Effects:*    Gain a new perspective, increased self-awareness.

# TAKEAWAYS

* By embracing movement and all movement that is possible in your body at any given moment, you have the ability to go from a place of avoidance to a place of abundance.

* When we invite in new perspectives through the body, we expand our perception in the mind.

* When we have a greater understanding of our own embodied feelings, we have a greater ability to express and manage them.

* When we move with more intention and attention, we are more conscientious of what influences our movements and how our movements impact the world around us.

# 8

# THE DANCE OF RESILIENCE

*Life isn't about waiting for the storm to pass,*
*it's about learning to dance in the rain.*
—VIVIAN GREENE

Life goes on whether we are ready for it or not. Resilience is a dance that everyone should learn in order to be more present and aware during or after a tragedy. Movement, being the core component of dance, is the foundation for accessing the ability to support and enhance our resilience.

Resilience resulting from body awareness and movement isn't a new concept. What I hope to add to the conversation is a focus on how certain movements support resilience. Overall we will be looking at how increasing your personal movement vocabulary, addressed in part I, leads to a more resilient body, which translates to a more resilient mind. Like any dance, resilience encompasses flexibility and adaptability, both of which can be facilitated through the body. Much like the variety and diversity inherent in different styles of dance, resilience is not necessarily a one-size-fits-all concept as it comes down to personal experience, culture, genetics, and environment.

## What Is Resilience?

Resilience is seen as the ability to recover quickly from challenges. Some would even say, to "bounce back." Psychologists define it as "the process of adapting well in the face of adversity, trauma, tragedy, threats, or significant sources of stress—such as family and relationship problems, serious health problems, or workplace and financial stressors."[1]

Recovery seems to suggest a return to a previous way of being or existing in the world. When we catch a cold, there is an assumption that we will return to our previous state of health and carry on with our "normal" functioning. Resilience, I believe, is more than recovery and it's not necessarily quick. It is an altered state that suggests that I'm becoming a new version of myself in order to adapt and thrive when faced with a challenging circumstance. Resilience is embodied recovery, but before we get into the embodiment of resilience, let's look at how it is influenced by the mind.

Mindset seems to play a huge role in resilience. Lolly Daskal, motivational speaker and executive leadership coach, discusses four common traits in resilient people:

- They are able to connect to their emotions.
- They don't listen to the negative voices in their heads.
- They know how to bounce back.
- They don't need to control everything.[2]

While I do not disagree with these, this approach is more cerebral and doesn't incorporate a physical aspect. A holistic (meaning treating the whole person) mind, body, and soul approach is imperative for building resilience. In their book, *Resilience: The Science of Mastering Life's Greatest Challenges,* Steven Southwick and Dennis Charney suggest ten ways to boost emotional resilience:

- Be optimistic
- Face your fears
- Have a moral compass

- Practice spirituality
- Get social support
- Have resilience role models
- Maintain physical fitness
- Keep your brain strong
- Be "cognitively flexible"
- Find meaning in what you do[3]

While these suggestions may be helpful for many people, different base levels of resilience must be taken into account. Simplified concepts like these are not enough for individuals who face more challenges in daily life. In a study published in *Frontiers in Behavioral Neuroscience,* researchers addressed how individuals achieve a sense of safety in a world that is anything but safe. Traumatic experiences highlighted included abuse in intimate relationships, refugee migration, and collective and historical trauma. Spirituality, connecting to "home," and social relationships were key to fostering resilience.[4] So it seems imperative that we find ways to support these.

The underlying principle that I see addressing all the above suggestions for building resilience is communication and connection with the body. Regular communication with the body can set the tone and potential for unleashing emotional resilience. When we are in our bodies, in the moment, we have the opportunity to access a sense of safety, whatever that means on an individual level. Even with regard to steps that encourage social support and mentoring, we can engage our bodies in certain dimensional planes to prep the mind for social engagement and outreach. Again, we must start with connection to self in order to feel safe enough to reach out. Remember back to chapter 5, where we explored the horizontal plane, where I embrace myself and spread that connection to the ones around me. For these and so many other reasons, body awareness and movement—including understanding how our movement impacts our outlook—directly supports and enhances our ability to become emotionally resilient. Looking at resilience as a dance, there are a few foundations needed for proficiency. I am a firm believer that everyone can dance; and with proper technique and practice, anyone can improve the skill. Resilience is no different.

> **BODY AWARE BREAK** Take a moment to "try on" recovery in your body. What does it look like to recover? Is it quick, slow, or sustained? Do you get a sense of bouncing back? What do you need in order to recover?

## Setting the Stage for the Dance

I want to introduce you to two key concepts that I use with all my clients. They are emotional temperature and emotional efficiency. Just like a body temperature, everyone has an emotional temperature, a psychological homeostasis that can be achieved through becoming more aware of our body and its internal landscape. We can learn to regulate our emotional temperature through awareness practices such as those involving breath, a body scan, and mindfulness. This entire book can be used as a way to manage your emotional temperature. When you are body aware you acquire an internal thermostat that regulates the variations in emotional energy you experience. Essentially, the more intense an emotion feels, the higher your emotional temperature. The lower or less connected you are to an emotion, the lower your emotional temperature is. Just like our body temperature, this naturally fluctuates throughout the day and depends on the presence of stressors. With any stress we have the ability to become dysregulated and overwhelmed or dissociated and checked out. Managing your emotional temperature is about regulation of body and mind.

Maintaining one's emotional temperature lends itself to emotional efficiency. Emotional efficiency refers to the expenditure of emotional energy. Much like a programmable thermostat in your home that conserves energy and money, when we are emotionally efficient, we conserve and preserve our mental health. Think for a moment of a time when you felt like your emotions were controlling you. All of your time and energy goes into that emotion, leaving little to no time for other activities. Don't we all want to devote time and energy to something of value or interest, rather than having it controlled or hijacked by anxiety, fear, anger, or other emotions? When we regulate our emotional temperatures we become more emotionally efficient people, freeing up our energy for the people, places, and activities that we want to focus on.

Another way I like to think of it is using a gas tank metaphor (or battery, for those of us who drive electric cars). Emotional efficiency means getting more emotional miles per gallon. We can build up reserves that allow us to manage stressors before they arise. Rather than risk running out of "gas" and getting stuck on the side of the road, being body aware supplies us with fuel or extra battery life for emotional emergencies. Sure you can send out some flares or call AAA, but wouldn't it feel better to have the tools to fill your own gas tank? I've experienced what it's like to run out of fuel emotionally and in my car, and I have found that having reserves makes a world of difference for my emotional and physical health.

So how do we regulate our emotional temperature to increase our emotional efficiency? At the heart of it is conditioning. It makes sense for people to emotionally condition themselves for uncomfortable situations, moments of confrontation, or difficult decisions. Conditioning is the process of training yourself to behave in a certain way or to accept certain situations and circumstances. We tend to focus on physical conditioning to limit injury and increase strength and endurance, but the same idea can be applied to emotional injury. This entire book is a guide to conditioning our emotional muscles. Again, through the body we create more awareness and the ability to manage life's stressors. There are things we can do every day to strengthen our emotional reserves, a stockpile of emotional energy to be used when needed at a later time and not just in the moment. Here are four strategies you should employ every day to build your emotional reserve tank.

BREATHING.   This includes noticing your breath as well as altering how you are breathing. Noticing your current breathing pattern, how much air you are taking in, and where the air is going is the first step to becoming aware of how well you are breathing. Zab Maboungou, a French-Congolese dancer, writer, and choreographer, says, "A body that doesn't know how to breathe doesn't know how to think."[5] Bringing more awareness and dimension to our breath enhances our ability to think and cope with our emotional landscape. When we increase the air capacity in our torso, it's like increasing our emotional gas tank, which means we get more "miles per gallon."

Revisiting the three dimensions from chapter 5, you can invite them into your breathwork. Sitting, standing, or lying down, imagine rays of light beaming out of the top of your head and down through the space between your legs. Breathe into this vertical dimension, lengthening as you exhale. Next, with your arms out to your side, imagine rays of light beaming out your fingertips. Breathe into this horizontal dimension, reaching as you exhale. Lastly, imagine a ray of light beaming through the center of your chest into the space in front of and behind you. Breathe into this sagittal dimension, recuperating as your exhale. You can also practice breathing into different parts of your body by visualizing the places you want the breath to travel. Support the body's ability to rest by extending the exhale as well as releasing the jaw.

Karina Kalilah, Rebirthing Breathwork facilitator and coach, offers this practice: Place your palms together, bring them in toward the chest, close your eyes if you feel so inclined, and take three generous breaths. The first breath signifies prayer for the Self. The second breath signifies a prayer for each other. The third breath signifies a prayer for the planet. I appreciate this practice as it reinforces the three dimensions and connection to Self, other, and the environment.

GROUNDING. This offers an opportunity to connect to the present moment. When we are in the present, we cannot dwell on the past or ruminate about the future. Grounding supports emotional regulation and conservation of emotional energy. Here are some grounding practices:

- Sitting or standing, plant your feet on the floor. Imagine your feet as roots connecting deep into the ground.

- Take a walk and notice every point of contact your feet have with the floor.

- Practice the 5-4-3-2-1 grounding exercise by calling to mind and body what you can see, touch, hear, smell, and taste.

**STRETCHING.** Stretching out makes us bigger. This is contradictory to how we move when we are in danger, physically and emotionally. We typically make ourselves smaller to decrease our visibility. Remember that pain, fear, anxiety, and stress in general constrict the body, making it harder to move. When we stretch, we increase the body's surface area as well as the internal space, allowing us to feel and move more. Creating more room in the body creates more space to process emotional stress. Additionally, when we stretch we create more opportunity for air capacity. Deeper breaths allow us to soften and drop into our bodies, circumventing the mind, which can keep us stuck in debilitating loops. Pandiculation in particular is a wonderful way to engage in this practice. This refers to the stretching action made when yawning, such as when we awake from sleep. The feeling of tension building in the body that then leads to a long stretch and release facilitates a progressive relaxation of the muscles, which not only creates extension in the body but also a loosening of sorts.

**ENGAGING IN MEANINGFUL MOVEMENT.** This, I believe, is most important! Meaningful movement is any movement that makes you feel good, energized, and connected. Meaningful movement is an authentic expression of your true self, which can make it more difficult to access if you are not used to accessing the Self in an authentic manner. It is not movement that is expected of you, forced on you, or performative. It is movement that fills up your cup, gives you energy, and lifts your spirits. This can be dancing in your living room, singing to your favorite song in the car, cooking for your family, sketching, journaling, or walking to a local coffee shop. Stop reserving certain times for physical activity. There are opportunities for meaningful movement everywhere. Deepak Chopra has been attributed as saying, "People need to know that they have all the tools within themselves."[6]

When your body is the toolbox, you have all the tools you need for healing all the time. In fact, *you* are all the tools you need.

## Moving toward Resilience

When we expand our movement repertoire—all the movement at our disposal—we increase our emotional resilience. I like to call this diversification of movement. When you diversify your movement, you broaden your body's ability to access a range of emotions, as well as your ability to manage them. Emilie Conrad, founder of the Continuum Movement, said, "The more capable a system [body] is the more it's able to manage whatever comes its way."[7] You may be familiar with the phrase "roll with the punches." This is what we are training the body to do in order to create a more resilient mind. We want the body to be able to move safely in as many ways as possible to access a sense of safety in as many ways as possible.

There are three elements that must be implemented into your movement to support resilience. These are playfulness, improvisation, and creativity. These support the diversification of movement as they encourage spontaneity, curiosity, and innovation. Let's explore each one.

While playfulness suggests feeling lighthearted and engaging in fun, it is so much more. Psychiatrist and play advocate Stuart Brown says, "Play is practice for the body." Play leads to a creative mindset as it is about breaking away from established habits and it encourages new perspectives, both of which are important to becoming body aware.[8] And if you remember from the last chapter, new perspectives come from moving in new ways. In the famous words of George Bernard Shaw, "We don't stop playing because we grow old, we grow old because we stop playing." Play provides an opportunity for us to use the imagination and to create something often reserved for the young but is actually necessary and accessible to all. Some of the most amazingly playful dance/movement therapy groups that I have led were not with children but with older adults in their nineties. The ability to play doesn't go away, but like everything else if we don't use it, we lose it.

With regard to our nervous systems, Lacy Alana, licensed clinical social worker and the creator of the Yes And Brain framework, suggests that play provides a "neural workout" through the alternating cues triggered when we move between danger and safety.[9] Think about a good old game of hide-and-seek. There is the safety of being hidden and the danger of being found. Learning to maneuver between these two dichotomies creates opportunity for emotional regulation. Suggestions for bringing more play into your life are playing games (e.g., board games, Pictionary, charades), imaginative role play, blowing bubbles, hopscotch, even visiting a neighborhood playground. These are all ways to support your own natural ability to play.

It has been said that "playfulness can be considered the mother that creates a state for both mindfulness and improvisation."[10] Improvisation dates back to 391 BC and is the spontaneous creation of ideas.[11] It encourages thinking and moving on the spot, being in the moment, and maybe even indulging impulsivity. This does not just mean signing up for a Second City class or an improv acting course; it's something that can be about creating opportunities for spontaneous movement in your life. Some examples are switching up a routine, walking or driving a different route, or switching directions.

For those of you who consider yourself movers or dancers, you might enjoy participating in Authentic Movement, an expressive improvisational movement practice. This practice is typically done in groups and allows a type of "free association of the body." Authentic Movement was founded in the 1950s by Mary Starks Whitehouse, a Jungian analyst residing in California.[12,13] Whitehouse recognized that simple unchanged movement reflected a person's true genuine self.[14] Alana says, "Improv is regulating for our lower brain, and invites us to feel deeply, respond to relational information, expand our window of tolerance, strengthen our social engagement system, and to better understand and rewrite the story of who we are and who we have the capacity to be."[15] Improvisation is an instrument that supports the development of creativity.

Creativity involves a novel form of behavior or novel idea. It is similar to improvisation in that it too involves breaking away from existing habits.[16] And it is related to play in that creativity is fostered through it. This is often why creativity is reserved for the young since as we age, our inclination to play seems to decline. There is a misconception that creativity peaks in our childhood, but that is not necessarily true. I think the fact is we don't leave time for creativity in our adulthood and like anything, what we don't use we lose. Creativity is a muscle that needs to be exercised and with regard to movement, trying new things is a must! Part of getting out of our comfort zone is moving in new ways.

**BODY AWARE BREAK** Here's an opportunity to bring new ways of moving into the body. Think of this as exercising your creative and improvisational muscles. Bring awareness to one of your hands. Attempt to move that hand and/or the fingers in five different ways. Repeat with the other hand. Try it with other parts of your body.

## Practice, Practice, Practice

How do we get better at a new skill? We practice! The dance of resilience is no different. We cannot necessarily wait for an instance to flex our resilience muscles. We must proactively engage in the diversification of movement.

We've taken the first two steps toward fostering resilience: learning how to take our emotional temperature and supporting resilience with playfulness, improvisation, and creativity. Now we move onto the next and perhaps hardest step: putting it all into practice. Prioritizing and making time to create more resilient bodies inherently leads to more resilient minds. Dr. Arielle Schwartz, clinical psychologist and author of *The Post-Traumatic Growth Guidebook,* has been quoted as saying, "Resilience ultimately allows us to embrace the unknown."[17] There is so much uncertainty in the world that we need all the help we can get to manage the inability to control everything. We can cope with the unknown by exposing our bodies to new, unusual, and uncomfortable movements, ultimately creating exposure to raw, underdeveloped, and underutilized emotions. Access to a wide range of emotions sets the stage for greater resilience, but we have to find opportunities to practice feeling more and moving differently.

That begins with moving our bodies in uncertain, uncomfortable, and new ways. Remember my daughter, the dance/movement therapist in training? When she was seven we had a marvelous conversation on how practicing feeling our emotions actually makes us more equipped to handle them. She asked, "Why would I want to practice feeling sad or frustrated?" To which I replied that while it might not feel good, when we allow ourselves to feel a full spectrum of emotions, we learn how to be with them. So next time you feel sad or frustrated, you can know what it feels like and what you need to help it move through you.

And for those of us who have spent time and energy avoiding certain emotions, this can make a world of difference. While I don't condone forcing yourself into emotionally compromising or unsafe situations just to "practice" feeling emotions, consider in what ways those emotions can be explored. Perhaps through a conversation with a friend, watching a movie or TV show, or reading a book where the characters themselves express those emotions.

So how can we practice and prioritize resilience from a body aware perspective? Let's begin with the spine. I find it vital to focus on the spine to support and enhance resilience. We know from previous chapters that accessing the spine taps into self-awareness. When we manipulate and engage the spine we create fluidity in the body. A fluid spine supports a resilient body, and a resilient body creates a resilient mind. This physical fluidity can support moving through life's challenges. A fluid spine makes for an emotionally healthy mind and body.

Dr. Candace Pert discovered neuropeptide receptors she calls "molecules of emotion," and while they are found throughout the body they are mainly found in the gut and spine. This suggests that manipulation of the spine impacts our emotions and it's quite possible that each position of the spine influences our emotional states, depending on what neuropeptides are present. Even small movements in the structure of the spine can contribute to the expression of different emotional chemistry. Consider that restricted motion in your spine lowers your emotional range. Furthermore, when the spine is distorted, it can keep us stuck in a certain emotion.[18]

This is why it is necessary from a mental health standpoint to find ways to support a healthy range of motion within your spine. A healthy range of motion translates to a healthy range of emotion. Here are some ways to encourage a wide spectrum of spinal mobility.

**CONTRACTING AND ARCHING THE SPINE:** Also known as Cat/Cow in yoga. This involves moving from rounding the back to arching the back. It is best to do this slowly, and rather than focusing solely on the spine, imagine it more as your head and tail trying to come together in each position. This can be done on all fours, standing, or in a seated position.

**ROLLING DOWN THROUGH THE SPINE:** Starting at the top of the spine, the base of the skull, slowly articulate through each vertebra like a zipper on a jacket. If you feel yourself skipping over them or going too fast, come back to the top and begin again. You can then reverse the motion, slowly coming back up to an upright position.

**RIB CAGE ISOLATIONS:** This may be a bit more advanced, but still worth practicing. This involves moving your rib cage independently from the rest of your torso. You can practice moving front and back, side to side, or in a circular motion.

**BODY ROLLS:** This involves rolling through the spine in a worm- or snake-like way. Starting either from the top of the head or tailbone, manipulate the spine in a fluid manner as if a wave in the ocean. You can play with different speeds and rhythms as well as the size of the movement. Can you involve your entire body?

Another way to diversify your movement, manage your emotions, and support resilience is through footwork. Footwork refers to quick or intricate movements of the feet and lower legs. This encourages agility in the body, not to mention coordination, mobility, and balance. There are lots of examples of "fancy footwork" available on the internet. I think of the jitterbug, stepping, tap dancing, hopscotch, double Dutch, and samba, to name a few.

Again, it's not simply about the steps, but the body's ability to move through different postures, positions, and patterns on and off the dance floor. You can even practice footwork by simply picking up the pace of a familiar workout. Put on some fast music and move your feet to the rhythm. Challenge your feet and how they move in any way possible to get out of your comfort zone. Make sure to slow things back down before moving on or starting another activity, as we want to encourage a regulated nervous system and not perpetuate speeding through life, but managing the fluctuations in the pace of life.

## A Quick Review

There are always notes given, feedback if you will, before the performance. So when it comes to the dance of resilience, here is the most important thing to know. Remember back to chapter 1, "Becoming Body Aware," when we were setting the foundation for this practice. I spoke about identifying your movement vocabulary, challenging your current movement, and expanding your movement repertoire. These are vital for creating a resilient body and mind. *A.C.E.* is a simple acronym you can use to remember:

Awareness of your current movement

Challenge your movement

Expand your movement

Integrating this acronym into your everyday life is the foundation of a body aware approach.

Once you have a good foundation, know the steps, and rehearse, the last piece is the performance—or in this case applying it to real-life situations. Integrating all of these tools into daily life is what this book is about.

Here's to creating more resilient bodies with a vast array of movement abilities. After all, it is these diverse movement capabilities that highlight and support the diversity in humankind.

## The Dance of Resilience in Motion

During an On the Move with PD group (a dance therapy support group dedicated to individuals and their caregivers impacted by Parkinson's disease), I invited the group to explore different movement qualities. Exploring *space* and *time*, the participants moved around the room, exploring big space and small space, quick time, and slow time, as well as all the elements in between. Halfway through there was an interesting shift. Many of the participants began standing up straighter, swinging their arms, and making eye contact with the other group members. As I brought this movement to a close, I invited them to reflect on this experience. Many of the members said that they usually engage in small movements in public because they are afraid of getting bumped into, losing their balance, and ultimately falling. This had not only limited their movement potential, but had begun to limit their social interaction. One participant said that she completely avoids public places because the fear and anxiety are too great. Exploring this movement in a safe, trusted environment allowed her to move through this place of fear and crippling anxiety. She quieted the doubts in her mind, faced her fear, and challenged herself to move in a different way. Exercising her resilience in that moment, she voiced her desire to go out in public and engage in hobbies and activities that she desperately craved.

## MOVEMENT RX: DAILY RESILIENCE DANCE

*Directions:*     If you are able and willing, you can lie down on the floor. This can also be done standing or sitting. Imagine that the floor or space around you is wet paint and that you must cover every inch of your body with it. Move in any way you can to "paint" your body. Pay attention to all the unusual ways you move in order to get into every nook and cranny. If lying on the floor is not possible or too uncomfortable, try using your hand and a hard surface like a table or desk. Move your hand in all directions to cover the entire surface of your hand with "paint."

    Once your entire body is "painted," imagine that the space around you is a blank canvas. Using your body as the "paintbrush," create a "painting" on the canvas. Again, focus on all the ways in which you can maneuver your body to "paint" the space around you.

*Dosage:*     Once a week or as needed.

*Side Effects:*     Increased movement ability, more creativity, enhanced resilience.

# TAKEAWAYS

* Regular communication with the body can set the tone and potential for unleashing emotional resilience.

* Just like a body temperature, everyone has an emotional temperature, a psychological homeostasis that can be achieved through becoming more aware of our body and its internal landscape.

* When we regulate our emotional temperatures, we become more emotionally efficient, freeing up our energy for the people, places, and things that we want to focus on.

* When your body is the toolbox, you have all the tools you need for healing all the time. In fact, *you* are all the tools you need to heal your emotional health.

* When you diversify your movement, you broaden your body's ability to access a range of emotions as well as your ability to emotionally manage them.

# 9

# DISABILITY AND DIVERSITY

*Disability is not something we overcome.*
*It's part of human diversity.*

—HABEN GIRMA, first deafblind graduate of Harvard Law School

All bodies are different from each other. This sounds like a simple statement, but even the somatic and movement worlds, which focus on movement diversity, still have a long way to go in accepting this basic fact. In this chapter, we'll be talking about the wide range of differences that people experience, both physically and cognitively, in their movement capabilities. When discussing movement diversity, we're talking about physical disability and neurodivergence as well as the individual patterns and behaviors that make each of us unique.

Let's break down some of these concepts. Disability is seen as a condition, physical or mental, that impedes a person's senses, movement, or activity. It is often interpreted as an inability to do what is seen as developmentally typical. Neurodivergence is a difference in mental or neurological function from what is perceived as typical or normal. Able-bodied refers to an individual without physical conditions that impact movement or activity. Even able-bodied people have body differences and diversity of movement. Not all disabilities are the same, and thus there's a huge range of diversity of movement among disabled folks too. Because disabled people have physical or cognitive conditions that can make life more difficult or require accommodations, they often learn to tune into their bodies more than able-bodied people do.

In my experience with clients, I have found that many individuals with memory impairments and neurodivergence have greater awareness and access to the present moment. Once again it is outsiders' judgments and assumptions that infer a lack of awareness simply because that person's reality may be different than their own. Language is not the only way to communicate. The body has something to say and will make its needs known.

When we see different ways of moving as unique attributes, they become strengths or exciting challenges. So regardless of our abilities or disabilities, how can we begin to see different ways of moving and being in our bodies as diversity and not just a difference? Remember that being body aware is not dependent on how well you verbally communicate what you are feeling and sensing but an ability to express it. It is imperative that we stop excluding people based on preconceived ideas around movement and start embracing all the ways individuals' movement patterns contribute to the diverse human experience. I believe it doesn't just come down to how much you move, but *how* you move—period.

> **BODY AWARE BREAK** Focus on a part of your body that physically feels limited. That could be a leg that you are sitting on, a joint that is achy, hands that have arthritis, sore muscles, or appendages with limited mobility. Pay attention to how it feels and any sensations that arise in that part. Listen to it. Give it a voice. What does it need?

The body doesn't judge. The mind judges and creates constructs of what the body "should" be doing, especially when others are doing it. We are influenced by what we see and hear from media, family, and constructed societal norms. The ego can be quick to speak for us, but communicating with the body and giving it the opportunity to move in any way possible is a path to empathy and understanding for ourselves and our fellow humans.

Judgment, specifically regarding movement, has been present in my line of work since I began as an intern. Especially when I worked with older adults, watching them either attempt to emulate my movements, witnessing caregivers move them according to how they "should" be moving, or disengage from movement altogether since they "can't do it." I have worked with younger individuals when caregivers place unrealistic expectations on how they should think, act, and move. When given the space, freedom, and creativity to exist in their bodies as they are—without judgment, expectation, or assumptions—movement happens naturally.

Stories of individuals with disabilities or different physical attributes performing difficult or "impossible" movements are often used as inspiration among able-bodied people, framed as instances of overcoming obstacles or defying odds. These stories aren't inspirational, though; they're simply stories of people achieving their personal potential. Movement in the presence of physical difference is not necessarily about overcoming anything. It's simply about moving, and as we've learned throughout this book, when we surrender to the dance of life, movement becomes the medicine we all need to soothe our emotional wounds. Movement in any and all forms is a universal remedy. It isn't about a specific way of moving but seeing movement as an extension of the Self. Just as every person is unique in their own way, so too is their movement—and that doesn't make them different or less than but part of the tapestry that creates diversity within the spectrum of humanity. We all have the ability to see diversity through movement and to encourage anyone to move for their own well-being.

## Seeing Diversity in Movement

No one moves exactly like you, and no one feels exactly what you feel in your body. Throughout this entire book we have looked for ways to increase awareness around our movements as well as ways to invite in new ways of moving. Beyond range of motion and flexibility, there are four steps to identifying and increasing the multiplicity of your movement:

1. **IDENTIFY HOW YOU CURRENTLY MOVE.** Just as we have been saying from part I of this book, awareness is the first step to creating change. This includes changing how we see our own movement abilities, which inherently impacts how we judge others. Taking time to notice your current movement ability provides a foundation for gratitude for what you have as well as empathy, understanding, and acceptance for how others move through the world.

This also goes for anyone you may be caring for who does not have the ability to make physical, environmental, or lifestyle changes for themselves. This could be a child, a student, or an elderly parent. Notice what movement you see in others, not to change it but to witness and even accept it. Become aware of how you feel when certain movements occur. Are you quick to silence them or stop them? Do you fear others will judge you for the actions of the people in your care? Remember you can look at movement as an expression of an unmet need. Begin to ask what those needs are and how they can be met, maybe even through movement. For example, a child having a tantrum in the middle of the grocery store might be enough to get even the calmest adult enraged or overwhelmed. Take a moment to identify your agenda (e.g., making it stop) and then create an opportunity to identify what the child needs. This can allow you to meet the child on their level, move with the child to another environment, or uncomfortably be the safe container for the child as they continue to experience intense emotional discharge.

2. **EXPLORE ALL THE WAYS MOVEMENT IS POSSIBLE FOR YOU.** This is another reminder to explore and embrace your potential for movement. This does not mean forcing movement onto your body, but inviting in what your body is capable of in each moment. For example, look at what postures are accessible in this moment. Intentionally deepen your breath, yawn, or stretch your body.

The same thing goes for those you live or interact with on a regular basis. Creating opportunities for them to explore all the movements they are capable of is vital for their mental health as well. Safety is of the utmost importance. If the environment is safe, or at least as safe as possible, then movement can be explored together. When I was working in nursing homes, even with all the staff present and clients seated, accidents happened. But I can say that the few times they occurred, the clients were calm, happy, and able to manage amid the fear or uncertainty because of how grounded and centered they were in their bodies. The sense of safety within spilled over to the sense of safety in the mind. The fear of consequences from moving should never stop movement from happening. Ensuring safety and security in one's environment, as much as possible, provides a much needed outlet for physical and emotional expression.

**3. FIND OPPORTUNITIES TO TRY MOVEMENT FROM A DIFFERENT PERSPECTIVE.** This can be from your own vantage point, moving into different postures or environments. This can also mean exposing yourself to movements with regard to different cultures. Keep in mind that culture is not just ethno-culture, but any group of people with similar interests. This can be physical abilities, races, religions, occupations, etc. How does movement differ between your office and the playground at the local park? Notice the different rhythms in people commuting to work versus relaxing at a local coffee shop. You may even notice different movement attributes within certain communities or neighborhoods. This can be seen in the hurried pace of people in a big city or the more relaxed stroll of people in a small beachside town.

Take the opportunity to mirror, not mimic or mock, but reflect someone else's movements. This is a key feature of a dance/movement therapist. Meeting others in their bodies—whether it is sitting on the same level, facing a similar direction, or embracing a similar posture—creates an embodied understanding a sense of being seen, validated, and supported on the most subconscious level.

**4. COMMIT TO LEARNING AND WITNESSING NEW WAYS OF MOVING.** This goes along with the previous step, but sets the intention for continued education. Once is not enough. We must commit to witnessing all forms of movement in order to embrace movement as diversity, not disability. This can include attending performances, traveling to places outside of your own cultural frame of reference, watching social media videos, or trying new dance forms or martial arts. Try to seek out teachers who carry an established lineage within their movement practice, as they are more likely to accurately represent the cultures from which the movements originated. You can often find information about an instructor's lineage on their studio's website.

## Disability and Diversity in Motion

I was contracted to run dance/movement therapy groups for an agency that provided programming for individuals with intellectual and developmental disabilities. I remember the first time I arrived to what had been described as the "lowest functioning" group. All members of the group were seated either in chairs or wheelchairs upon my arrival. It was clear that participants were expected to follow my lead, so when I encouraged the participants to move in their own way, it was met with a little skepticism. One gentleman in particular was mobile and discouraged from wandering about, since his seizure disorder could lead to falling and sustaining a head injury. I remember his posture being quite constricted. He never raised his arms above his shoulders and his movements were very repetitive. He also was unable to stay in one place for very long, was fixated on lunch that was hours away, and engaged very little with others during our session.

On my third visit I began the group as always, greeting each participant around the room, inviting them to engage in a gentle body warm-up to familiar music, and eventually creating opportunity for social dance among the staff and participants. During the social dance, this gentleman sought me out. I encouraged the staff to allow this to happen. He grabbed my hands and interlaced his fingers with mine bringing them up to about chest level. He began swaying side to side, almost losing his balance on one leg before shifting to the other. We moved together, in sync, making eye contact and smiling. He then began to stretch his arms up over his head and muttered his name, introducing himself. While stretching our arms up, I acknowledged his presence, introduced myself, and thanked him for dancing with me. He let go of my hands and connected with another person, a staff member who replicated the same thing. This happened with as many people as he could engage with, some even sitting down. The connection, energy, and joy sparked around the room was tangible.

On my fourth visit, I noticed another participant sitting in a chair with his back against the wall. During an impromptu dance party, his feet tapped to the beat of the music and his hands clapped. I noticed as staff members approached him to engage or dance with him, he would turn his head, drop his gaze, and stop moving. As the person walked away he would resume. I decided to approach him, but crouched down next to him side by side. I began mirroring his movements and rhythm. He turned his head toward me, smiled, and gave me a hug.

## MOVEMENT RX: MOVEMENT GREETINGS

*Description:*   Identify and try out five different ways to say hello with your body.

Identify and try out five different ways to say goodbye with your body.

*Dosage:*   Use a different salutation with each person you meet within a week.

*Side Effects:*   Greater range of expression; diverse perspectives.

## TAKEAWAYS

* The body doesn't judge.

* Movement in the presence of physical differences is not always about overcoming anything but about the right to achieve one's potential.

* When we surrender to the dance of life, movement becomes the medicine we all need to soothe our emotional wounds.

* Just as every person is unique in their own way, so too is their movement, and that doesn't make them different or less than, but part of the tapestry that creates diversity within the spectrum of humanity.

# 10

# PUTTING IT INTO PRACTICE

*Knowledge is of no value unless you put it into practice.*
—ANTON CHEKHOV, Russian dramatist

If you are anything like me, you read a book—maybe even highlight the important parts you want to remember, and recommend it to others; but within a few weeks or months the information slips away, replaced by the next book, article, or information source. I find that unless I practice and integrate the knowledge into my daily life, it becomes a faint memory of something I intended to do but couldn't figure out how to implement.

The last thing I want this book to become is a distant memory. The whole point is that readers walk away with a new way of being in the world and in their bodies. This section is dedicated to real-life scenarios and situations from my personal experience as well as from years of being a therapist.

## Movement as a Metaphor

I love using metaphors in my therapy sessions. They can provide visuals for difficult concepts. Dr. Kathlyn Hendricks asks the question, "How can a concept be translated into movement?"[1] This is something I ask myself every day. I find it challenging and exciting to find ways that movement supports different ideas. It makes me feel like a detective, trying to figure out the best way, in the moment, to figure out how to connect mind and body. For example, "taking a stance" on a political issue when put into the body can allow us to figure out literally where we stand on the issue. Literally "putting your foot down" invites in an embodied awareness of what happens when you set a boundary. And "tiptoeing" around a subject when explored through movement can highlight what it feels like when we avoid an issue.

Anytime you are unsure of what you are feeling is a time to go into the body to try on what that feels like and how moving it can enhance your perspective or create a new level of awareness. The following phrases and scenarios are not meant to be a model for what you have to do, but rather a guideline for how you can embrace a body aware approach in everyday life. Let's begin with some common phrases or comments that we may hear or say in our daily lives.

## "You Look Tired"

Have you ever been on the receiving end of the comment, "You look tired?" Perhaps you have said it to someone or even thought it as you caught a glimpse of your reflection. My initial thought to this comment is, "Gee, thanks!" But on further introspection, I have begun to ask myself, "What about my body or movement suggests I am tired?" Maybe I am and I don't even realize it. My body is obviously talking and something about it might suggest that I am in need of rest. Keep in mind that what others see as "tired" could be a projection of how they feel or what they see in themselves.

Notice that we are often defensive when others point out something other than how great we look. Perhaps others can be the mirror we are afraid to look into. Take this moment to check in with your body and mind to see if there is any sense of fatigue. While you may not have the ability to sleep or even lie down, there are simple movements you can do to increase your energy, focus, and attention. Try rubbing your hands together and then reaching your arms up toward the sky. Shake out your hands and bounce or bend your knees. Take three short inhales through your nose and then exhale through your mouth, also known as "Bunny Breath." The idea is to energize the body and invigorate the mind using movement-centered approaches that connect your body and mind to the present moment.

If you are in fact fatigued, this is the time to prioritize rest. So often rest is seen as a sign of being unproductive, lazy, or unmotivated. For an anxious mind, as an example, rest can be productive. When stillness and silence welcome worry, rest can seem impossible. Getting to a place where we don't have to fill our time with busyness offers an opportunity for recuperation. So the next time someone mentions that you look tired could be the chance for you to reconnect mind and body and prioritize rest and emotional recovery.

## "You're Being Too Sensitive" or "You Are So Sensitive"

I heard this phrase a lot growing up, and I hear it a lot in sessions with clients. *Sensitive* usually corresponds to being emotional or showing emotions. Notice what you feel when someone says this to you. Where do you connect to sensitivity and how does your body move when feeling emotional? Are you more inclined to express yourself or less inclined? Whatever you need to express is valid and just because someone cannot handle those emotions themselves doesn't mean you shouldn't be allowed to experience them. Find a way to express these feelings. This may be through movement, journaling, drawing, listening to or playing music. It is not about eliminating feelings, thoughts, and emotions. It is about working and *moving* through them.

Keep in mind that there is also judgment with this phrase. It is someone else's perception of your emotional status. How do you manage criticism? Are you the constant receiver of criticism by a family member? When we are made to feel criticized for experiencing emotions, we begin to minimize them and even deny we have them. This is a good opportunity to notice what your body does when the mind denies feelings and emotions. Do you shrug it off, push it down, bottle it up? All of these show up in the body. Allowing yourself to notice what is happening creates space to counterbalance these effects.

Notice next time how the presence or even just the thought of a person who offers criticism may impact your body posture. Some people close in and become smaller, while others may overcompensate by puffing out their chest and creating a larger-than-life posture. What do you notice, and how does it impact your mental health or ability to be present? It can be helpful to engage in movements that promote the opposite of what your body is inclined to do. This is not to suggest jumping into it, but in order to not perpetuate ingrained habits, begin to explore what it would look or feel like to bring polarities into your movement. Feel yourself shrinking or overextending? Come back to center aligning your spine and focusing on self-awareness. This allows you to focus on your personal thoughts and beliefs and disengage from the judgment of others.

## "I'm Sorry"

If this is in your daily vocabulary, you will know by how your body reacted when you read this heading. It is definitely familiar to me. These two words have been so ingrained in many of us. It was modeled for me, and even when I made an effort to change my vocabulary so as not to pass it down to my children, it still crept into their language as a way to quickly make others feel more comfortable. While apologizing is important if you have caused harm or hurt someone, saying sorry, or assuming fault, is not necessary in most situations.

When I stopped automatically saying sorry, I began to reflect on the situation and ask myself, "What happened to make me feel sorry?" Let me offer this example. I noticed that when I said sorry for bumping into someone on the sidewalk or in the mall, I became smaller; my torso closed in and my gaze often fell. My words said, "Sorry," but my body said, "I am in the way and others have more of a right to be here than I do." When I began to notice this response, not only did I stop saying sorry, but I didn't apologize for taking up space. Rather I respectfully excused my lack of spatial awareness and reinforced my right to be there simply by shifting my body and owning my boundaries. While it is a valuable lesson to learn to acknowledge and take responsibility for harm we may cause, when we notice what our bodies do it allows us to understand what we need while we hold remorse, guilt, sorrow, or shame.

The next time you say sorry, notice how your body moves. Do you find yourself shrinking or growing? Is there a sarcastic tone or a sincere apology? How you move in relation to your apology can mean the difference between reinforcing your own lack of self-worth and taking responsibility and embracing ownership for something you did.

## "Running Out of Patience"

This may be something you say to a child or experience while waiting longer for something than you expected. Again, notice what is happening in your body as your patience "runs" low. There may be a constricting in your torso, crossing of the arms, tapping of the feet, or exaggerated affect like rolling eyes, clenched jaw, maybe even grunting or groaning. If I am waiting in line somewhere and it hasn't moved, I notice that I begin to shift my weight from side to side and look around. This signals to me that my patience is being challenged. I wasn't blessed in the patience department, so I have many opportunities to work on this. I may have no control over how quickly the line moves, but I do have the ability to manage my emotions as I wait. Why am I in such a rush? Where else would I rather be? What else could I be doing? These are all questions that allow me to understand why I might not want to be standing around. I bring awareness to the present moment by engaging the senses. Try identifying five things you can see, four things you can hear, three things you can touch, two things you can smell, and one thing you can taste.

Consider what emotions are in abundance as your patience runs low. In my own experience, patience is a combination of the elements of space and time. When both feel restricted or out of my control, I begin to lose the ability to be in the moment. I anticipate the future or dwell on the time wasted. What elements do you feel present? Finding ways to indulge these elements, like taking up space by stretching or breathing or intentionally slowing down your movement can make a world of difference and actually build those emotional reserves discussed in chapter 8.

## "Pull Yourself Together"

This phrase suggests that you are falling apart, which emotionally may feel true, but physically isn't entirely logical. This is most often reflected in our thoughts or speech, but remember that our body is also displaying signs of overwhelm. Notice what parts of your body are held, bound, or tight and what parts are loose, disconnected, or distracted. What is your posture like in this moment?

You can use your body to reinforce what you want to feel in your mind. This is the perfect opportunity to find your spine. Stack those knees, hips, and shoulders to align them so you can feel your body coming together from the inside. Consider also engaging in a pulling motion. Pull an imaginary rope toward you. Reach for something you imagine really wanting or needing and pull it into your body.

You can place your palms against a wall while standing or move to the floor on all fours, knees and palms. Find a neutral spine and relax your shoulder blades. You will feel your chest sink toward the floor and your shoulder blades kiss. Now push your shoulder blades away from each other as your chest moves away from the floor and lengthen your spine. This is another variation of pulling yourself together as you feel your spine align. Recuperate in Child's Pose and breathe.

## "Relax" or "Calm Down"

This phrase always makes me laugh a little because it typically accomplishes the exact opposite of what is intended. I used to get this a lot at the doctor's office while I was silently freaking out. I can't even tell you how many times I heard it from the nurses in Labor and Delivery while having my first child. Hearing the phrase "calm down" only reinforced that I wasn't calm, and it made me feel ashamed or as if something was wrong with me. I also noticed that I became very talkative; my speech pattern inherently matched the pace of my thoughts until I became so overwhelmed that I couldn't speak fast enough, so I froze and became silent.

When I stopped focusing on the words and started paying attention to how my body was not calm or relaxed, I was able to truly listen to what my body was saying. Paying attention to the parts of your body that are not relaxed or calm allows you to find ways to listen. This is the first step in managing the emotions that hinder or prevent us from calming down.

My silence became a sign to me of my rising emotional temperature. When I became silent I knew I had an emotional fever. One way I found to bring the fever down was to laugh. When I laughed it brought in all the movement qualities that my body was lacking. I became lighter and looser as opposed to heavy, tight, and bound. I would encourage someone to tell me a joke or a funny anecdote and immediately my body shifted. Now I go so far as to request a certain nurse when I go for my checkups or annual exams because my body and mind associate positive interactions with these people.

Think of an overactive or really excited child. The go-to directive is often "sit down!" This again is counterproductive because the body is not able to be still; it needs more movement to find a natural way to recuperate. Engaging in larger, more active movements can allow the child to modulate their own energy. This can look like running in place, taking a lap around a school gym, or jumping/bouncing. This empowers the child to organically find a way to calm down instead of being forced into it.

## "Get Over It," "Move On," or "Let It Go"

These are all variations of the same thing: a need to hold on. The art of letting go is in the ability to recognize what you are trying to hold onto or maintain. So again, we look to represent holding on in the body in order to find a way to somatically let go.

Pay attention to what happens in your body when being forced to or coerced into letting go. The mind will not be able to let go of something when the body is still holding onto it. When we acknowledge what it looks or feels like as we hold onto something or someone, we can begin to understand what is needed to let go. Then we can begin to move through the difficult emotions that come up.

If someone is telling you to "move on," it can be a reflection of their discomfort in watching you flounder or continue to make the same decisions expecting different results. This is when working with an unbiased professional can help you identify what has a hold over you, because once you can identify what you think you cannot be without, you can begin to focus on what it is you really need.

## "Dance Like No One's Watching"

While I have been known to use this phrase myself I, do see some limitations. First, why limit it to dance? I say, "Move like no one's watching." Second, there is an assumption that we are only free to move when eyes are not on us: but for some, movement is just as inaccessible. It is their own internal judgment that prevents many people from moving through the world unapologetically.

It is important to move without fear of judgment—period. Notice what happens in your body when just the thought of moving in front of others comes to mind. This might even be public speaking. I'm not suggesting that you join a flash mob, but there is value in finding ways to move in public. This might include walking through an airport, attending a concert, or taking an exercise or dance class at a local park district. Take time to check in with your body and notice how you move in these situations. The point is to tap into a sense of freedom in your body and mind. What would it look and feel like to move without judgment? When was the last time that was even possible?

———

Now, let's look at some common situations or scenarios that we encounter on a regular basis. Many of these we experience on autopilot and have no idea how they are impacting our bodies. Keep in mind that nothing is meant to be a quick fix but rather an opportunity to change the way you manage your reactions during these situations.

## Unrecognized Gestures

Have you ever held the door for someone, only to have it go unrecognized? Maybe this doesn't bother you, but this used to enrage me. I would scornfully stomp off in a bad mood and scorn the way the world's morals have plummeted. I even went so far as to loudly say, "You're welcome!"

I grew tired of caring so much about this and went into my body to see what was going on. I noticed in my body that I was looking for gratitude and wanted to be recognized for a good deed. When that went unnoticed I felt betrayed, ignored, and invisible. This was reflected in how I felt when someone else held doors for me. I wanted to acknowledge them and show my gratitude. So naturally when it wasn't reciprocated, I internalized it and felt angry.

Now, I consider how it makes me feel to do something for someone else regardless of their response. A "thank you" is icing on the cake. Now I can walk away confidently knowing that my movement (holding the door for someone) is an extension of my caring nature and not fishing for gratitude from a stranger. I hold my head up and stand firm in my chivalrous gesture. And if someone doesn't notice it, it is simply because they aren't aware, not because they are trying to intentionally hurt my feelings. Maybe now as they walk through the door, I'll give them this book! Seriously, though, it is often a testament to how unaware we are and how accustomed we are to operating on autopilot, not the disinterest or inability to show gratitude.

## Dichotomous Thinking

Also known as binary or black-and-white thinking, this often entails an all-or-nothing outlook on life. This is very common especially with younger individuals, but also with people who have experienced trauma. We can be forced to choose between one or the other, when in reality there is quite a large spectrum. The body is typically very rigid in terms of binary thinking, meaning there are only two ways of doing something, right or wrong, safe or unsafe, open or closed. When we embrace the movement spectrum, the gray area—so to speak, our ability to see options and choices increases. We can find out-of-the-box ways to problem-solve and critically think in order to ease our suffering.

Try identifying through the body the polarities that exist in your current way of thinking. What are the qualities present in the movement? Find a way to move along the spectrum or flow between the two polarities. As you try this on, notice what happens to your thought process.

## Road Rage

While I'm not one to exhibit this, I have definitely witnessed it and been on the receiving end of it. There are so many body cues that must be present prior to exhibiting full-on road rage. Think of your car and the way you drive it as an extension of your emotional condition. Again, while this is not set in stone or scientifically proven, it is my perspective and experience. People who are emotionally hypo-aroused drive slower, while those who are hyper-aroused drive faster. Both can be dangerous, and both lack the same thing: the awareness that how you feel is influencing how you are driving.

It is to your benefit, as well as the safety of those you share the road with, for you to notice how your body is carrying your emotional baggage even while driving. How does your lack of awareness hinder your ability to operate heavy machinery? I strongly believe there is a correlation between our decreased embodiment and increased vehicular accidents. What is distracting you from being fully present while behind the wheel, and what can you do to increase your ability to be in the moment?

I love to drive by myself. It helps me think, clear my head, and just be in the moment. So when I notice that I'm flustered behind the wheel or heavier on the gas pedal, it is an opportunity for me to literally slow down. I decelerate the car to decelerate my mind. Taking my foot off the gas pedal or just easing the tension and pressure in my foot allows me to lighten the tension in my body. I sit back into my seat or adjust my posture and bring attention to what is causing this emotional discharge. While I might not be able to address the underlying cause immediately, I can be proactive and address how it is impacting my current physical and emotional state.

## Feeling Stuck

This is a common occurrence and the preface for much of this book. Keep in mind that feeling stuck can also be experienced as feeling frozen, emotionally and physically. When do you feel stuck, and how does your body perpetuate this? I personally notice a correlation between feeling stuck and a lack of creative outlets. Dance for me helps to get my creative juices flowing, but due to schedules and responsibilities, I am not always able to take a dance class. This leads to restriction in my expressive outlets—which inevitably leads to more stress, overwhelm, and emotional stagnation.

The best example I can think of is the COVID-19 pandemic. Not only did many of us go into lockdown, but so much of our world went virtual. Using the example of dance classes specifically, I attempted to dance on Zoom in the privacy of my home, but it just didn't provide the outlet I needed. In fact, I noticed that it made me more anxious and uptight. This is when I made a real effort to look for other ways to move through this difficult time. When the weather permitted, I got outside. I took long walks free from technology so I could focus on being in the moment. Feeling stuck, for some, is about a lack of connection—to self and to others. Finding ways to connect to yourself through breath, spinal modulation, and exploring the dimensions of movement discussed in chapter 5, are all ways to reinforce movement when we feel immobile or stuck.

Consider that when we cannot move in the ways we want to, we often stop moving. If I cannot run, then I just won't exercise. This denies ourselves the emotional outlet our bodies and minds need. It is imperative to find other ways to move in order to let our thoughts, feelings, and emotions run freely.

Remember that feeling stuck is not just mental but physical. Notice what parts of your body are held, bound, constrained, and unmotivated.

Look for any and all ways that movement is possible, no matter how small it may be.

## Balancing Act

Multitasking or trying to manage multiple things at once can be overwhelming, to say the least. We fool ourselves into thinking we are balancing these tasks, but that is a façade. When we multitask we end up doing many different things at half capacity and this can go hand-in-hand with feeling stuck, especially if trying to balance everything leads to immobilization. Yes, trying to balance can lead to restricted movement because we are so focused on controlling or holding things in place that the slightest movement can lead to the feeling that everything will drop. With regard to the pandemic example above, I recognized that my lack of dance in particular was contributing to my feeling stuck. I coupled that with my overwhelming need to juggle motherhood, client caseload, e-learning, etc., and found myself in my basement one day sitting with my daughter who was trying to juggle balls. She was learning this, or rather was encouraged to try it, in her PE Zoom class. A light bulb came on for me. I taught myself over the next few weeks to juggle. Not only did it allow me to use my brain, tap into my creativity, and move, but it helped me literally embody the juggling act that was my life. Dropping the ball— literally—reinforced that dropping the ball in life was not only unavoidable, but it wasn't the end of the world. I could pick up those balls and try again. Furthermore, it was fun and a good challenge.

So what does it look like for you when you lack balance or are holding on for dear life with the fear that you will fall or fail? Imagine what it would feel and look like in your body to find stability, equilibrium, and harmony.

## Finding Your Voice

Speaking up, verbalizing your needs, and just being able to voice a concern or opinion can be a huge challenge, especially when you have been conditioned to feel like your voice doesn't matter. When I have difficulty speaking up, I find it helpful to notice where I feel what I need or want to say. While many people identify their throat or neck, you might be surprised to find that it is in your abdomen, hips, or maybe even your hands. Identifying where your voice originates can help you support and validate your own need to be heard. Additionally, once you "find" your voice, you can explore ways of expressing it and making it heard.

## Standing Up for Yourself

This can be an extension of finding your voice. So often we don't have access to our own self-worth or value, which makes it even harder to voice what we need. What does it look like to stand up for yourself? What do you need in order to do that? Usually it requires support, which we may not have from others. So this becomes about finding your own support. This is when a wall and the floor can come in very handy. Use the walls or floors of your room, hallways, or houses to find support. How does it feel when you have support? What can you do for yourself when you have the support you need?

Once you have felt or accessed support, notice how it feels to stand on your own. Find different ways to stand on your feet. This can begin with sitting or lying down while feeling your feet on the floor. What happens as you begin to increase your self-awareness through connection to the supportive structures in your environment?

## Social and Peer Pressure

No one is exempt from this. The difference is how connected you are to yourself and your ability to stand in those values, even when it contradicts those around you. What does pressure feel like in your body? Finding ways to identify with it and move it or release it can make a big difference in standing your ground or succumbing to it.

Notice what you need in order to not give into pressure. Perhaps support, connection, community, or a welcoming environment or space to call your own. What enables you to give in to the pressure? You may be able to identify a breaking point, and what happens in the body leading up to that point can allow you to manage it as it arises.

## Transitions

This could be a chapter in itself. Transitions are one of the top three reasons most clients see me. Whether it is graduating college, becoming a parent, or "adulting," life is one big transition. When we deny the body's role in these transitions, it becomes much harder to maneuver through them. The mind replays what the body displays. If your body is displaying anxiety, discomfort, or uncertainty, that will show up in your thoughts and influence your ability to make a transition.

Keep in mind that how quickly you move through a transition isn't always about your ability to adapt but can be a reflection of your inability to slow down, veer from the course, or sit in discomfort. Identify two different markers in your current environment. Assign one as point A and the other as point B. Give yourself the opportunity to move back and forth as efficiently and inefficiently as possible. Notice what changes. Which one is more familiar? Which experience do you play out in everyday life?

Another practice is transitioning from one room to the next in your home. Notice what happens in your body. Do you move in certain ways depending on what room you are in? What about when you transition from indoors to outdoors, your home to someone else's home, or from home to work or school? You have the opportunity to embrace and practice transitions every day. Notice where they already exist in your life and make a point to engage your body.

## Getting Things Done

I am a list maker. I love the satisfaction of crossing something off my to-do list. For the longest time, I thought the more I got done in one day, the better I would feel, but it just left me feeling exhausted and looking for the next set of things that needed to be done.

What I realized is that keeping busy was a tool for avoidance. Yes, it felt good to accomplish tasks, but it was also a way for me to not pay attention to certain feelings. Here's a thought: we can slow down to do more. Additionally, the quality of the task or work goes up. It goes back to the old saying, "Quality over quantity." That can be said for movement. It is not always about how much or how often you move, it is also about the quality of the movement.

Take time to slow your movements down. This doesn't mean moving in slow motion necessarily but paying attention to how you move, and if it is rushed or hurried, then change the pace. Slow down your breathing or your walking, and notice how it impacts the pace of thoughts swimming around your mind.

## Rest

This is a triggering word for some people, as the thought of it alone can bring on anxiety. The truth is everyone needs rest. Keep in mind that we recharge our cell phones and other electronic devices to the point that we don't leave the house without backup chargers. But when it comes to our own brains and bodies, we often rely on caffeine and sleeping pills.

Take time to notice what prevents your mind from resting and see if it is possible to introduce that into the body. For example, if I have trouble winding down after a taxing day and my mind is still swirling, I use this opportunity to find stability in my body. I might begin by moving in a swirling motion to symbolize what I feel in my mind. I will then allow my body to gradually shift into a calmer rhythm. This can be done on a smaller scale using just your hands, your feet, or a guided imagery using only your imagination.

## Applications for Parenting

Everything in this book is adaptable for children. There are many exercises I began using with my own kids when they were toddlers. It is never too early to start good mind-body hygiene. There is an iconic 1972 slogan from the United Negro College Fund that says, "The mind is a terrible thing to waste." I believe the mind-body connection is a terrible thing to waste. When we embrace it as parents we can hone our intuition, better support our children's experiences, be more mindful of when we are pushing our own agenda, and model for our kids what it looks like to be responsible for our own emotions.

You might be surprised at how easily kids grasp the concepts in this book, as they have less experience with overriding their bodies' needs. They live in their emotions and crave creative ways to express themselves. If you are a parent who struggles to find effective coping strategies for your children's emotional well-being, I encourage you to look at the creative arts therapies. They are for all ages, but extremely accessible for children, who are inherently connected to their creativity.

We also can be better children ourselves. We can recognize the difference between what we need and what our parents think we need. We can learn to be responsible adults and find security in being our own person with our own beliefs, thoughts, and emotions. Movement is a necessary way to re-parent the inner child who was minimized or neglected.

---

This is by no means an exhaustive list, but a jumping-off point for you to implement body wisdom and awareness into everyday scenarios. Once again it is not about waiting for an opportunity to move, but recognizing all the ways we can use our movement to support our current situations. I recognize that these aforementioned scenarios can also be interpreted in other ways. I encourage you to find your own metaphors and meanings in your movements. At the very least begin to bring your body into these conversations.

Use every opportunity as a chance to practice listening to your body. If you are waiting to make changes, you need not wait any longer. Simply begin to pay attention to what is happening in your body right now. That is all you need to begin your path to healing, wellness, and resilience. You have all the tools you could possibly need to move your way toward the life you deserve.

# CONCLUSION

I began this book by asking a simple question: "How are you moving today?" This book has provided you with all the tools and resources to answer that question and to continue exploring how that very question has everything to do with who you are and how you move through life, physically and emotionally. Because at the end of the day it isn't just *how much* you move, but *how* you move that matters. This is by no means an end; this is the beginning. This is where you take the knowledge and apply it to your life. You can revisit any part of this book anytime you need a reminder of how you already have all the tools you need inside of you.

I may have failed to mention two major side effects from reading this book. First, you will feel more and you will feel everything deeply. When we allow ourselves to be more vulnerable in a safe and healthy way, we open ourselves up to profound feeling. Many of my clients express feeling intense emotions during our journeys together. However, this isn't necessarily perceived as negative, but on the contrary, life-affirming and life-giving. For the first time, many of them are able to consciously allow emotions in and to be with them. The more you allow yourself to identify and be with your emotions, the more you will understand why they are present and how to manage them.

Here's the thing: when you have closed off your body and mind to feeling, allowing yourself to feel again can be like opening the floodgates. You must remember two things. One is that this is a sign of healing. In the words of Dr. Caroline Leaf, author of *Cleaning up Your Mental Mess: 5 Simple, Scientifically Proven Steps to Reduce Anxiety, Stress, and Toxic Thinking,* "When you start to feel intensely, know you are healing immensely."[1] Two is that when you start to feel deeply, the body is where you will find support as well as an outlet for the emotions. The point of bringing the body into awareness is to support your mental health. That is the piece

I truly believe has been missing from mainstream mental health conversations. It is not just about exercising and meditating. We must recognize what our bodies are holding in order to release it so we do not continue to repeat the same patterns.

It is important to note that with change—even positive change—grief is inevitable. As we welcome a new way of being in the world, we say goodbye to the old habits, patterns, and paradigms that shaped our identity. Stepping into a stronger, healthier, and more centered you still means grieving the loss of the you that previously existed for so many years. Making space to process this grief in the body is ultimately what will allow the mind to move through it.

Second, you will gain a stronger sense of identity by understanding more about yourself, your needs, your boundaries, and your abilities. Identity isn't defined by movement placed onto the body, but by movement from inside the body, and it must come from a sense of being in the body. When your identity is defined by your talent or career, achievements and accomplishments are everything; and when they are threatened, so is your very existence. It becomes easy to lose ourselves when we don't perform up to our standards or the expectations of others. Befriending your body can mean the difference between being disappointed and feeling like a disappointment. Your body is constant, while skill, talent, or occupation can be fleeting, environmental, or circumstantial, so it is in your best interest to use your body and mind to build a safe supportive connection that is yours regardless of your success, wealth, or reputation.

This book provides a framework that focuses on being *pro*active, not *re*active. When we take the time to connect to our bodies, we can recognize the range left on our emotional gas tank and choose how far we can go with the emotional reserves we have. This isn't to say that you will never react, but the time you spend reacting and the recovery time thereafter will lessen. Additionally, based on your range you can choose how and when to engage in situations. You wouldn't drive a hundred miles if you only had less than a gallon of gas left in the tank, so why overextend yourself by taking on more than your emotional range can handle? This is the power of becoming body aware, taking charge of your emotional health by embracing the body that influences it.

Movement alone does not guarantee positive mental health. Otherwise, professional athletes, artists, and performers would be the gold standard when it comes to mental health, and we know that is not always the case. While strength corresponds to mind and body, without the frequent dialogue between them and the ability to check in with the load on both, the mind can be quick to override the body's needs. We can push through, overexert, and burn out. This book is a guide to living your best life. Not by adopting a positive outlook but by adopting a way to move through everything life throws at you, and understanding how the way you move during challenging times is just as—if not more—important than the way you move when things feel easy.

It has been a challenge and a joy to share this information with you. I wish you continued support, curiosity, and patience for your healing journey. I believe everyone deserves to feel their emotions without fear of judgment or punishment. May we all find ways to express ourselves through movement while holding the space to honor what that movement feels like and what it means on a personal level. It is my hope that this book has moved you, mind, body, and soul, and I thank you for moving with me.

# Acknowledgments

This book would not have been possible without the following people, and to them I am eternally grateful. While I am grateful to all my dance teachers and educators along the way, there is a special place in my heart for Dr. Rusti Brandman, Associate Professor Emeritus of Dance at the University of Florida. Rusti, you were the first person to ever utter the words *dance/movement therapy* to me. Your guidance and direction literally brought me to where I am today. I cannot even begin to thank you enough for your insight and intuition about merging my passions of psychology and dance.

Thank you to Kris Larsen and Nikki Levine for your years of personal and professional support. I have always tried to model my abilities as a therapist around your practices. The client experiences in this book were in large part due to your guidance, as you two have collectively become the clinical voice in my mind and body.

Thank you to Leslie Levine, not only for creating the title, but for planting the seed for this book in my mind and body. You were the first mentor and guide who challenged me to find my voice and share my story. Your willingness to chat about my vision meant the world to me. Your guidance and direction from an author's perspective was invaluable and a huge reason this book came to fruition.

Thank you to Rea Frey for getting the ball rolling. Without your drive, support, and encouragement, this book still would be just a dream. Your professionalism, kindhearted nature, and business-savvy wit was exactly what I needed to steer this project in the right direction. Your candid and honest introduction into the literary world kept me grounded and optimistic. You are a treasure, and I am so glad our paths crossed.

Thank you to my literary agent, Linda Konner, for not only believing in my vision but agreeing to take on this project. From your honest feedback to your encouragement through the acquisition process, I am so glad to have your knowledge, fierceness, and years of expertise on my side. Without you I would not have the next person to thank.

Shayna Keyles, my editor and fellow Jersey girl. Everything from your insight and expertise to your support and enthusiasm has made this process a delight. I couldn't imagine a better working relationship. Thank you for bringing me into North Atlantic Books, to whom I am also grateful. Your warm welcome into the NAB family has allowed me to see that this is where my book was meant to be. It is an honor to be in the company of the amazing authors you represent.

Thank you to my friends and colleagues, Jesse, Azizi, Becky, and Donna, who provided feedback on the manuscript and supported it (and me) in its earliest phases. Your assistance made this book come to life.

Thank you to Dr. Nicole LePera. Your willingness to support this book in addition to your commitment to holistic approaches to mental health are commendable. I am forever grateful to you for answering my direct message on Instagram, and I look forward to witnessing all the future has in store for you.

To Amber Gray, thank you for your guidance on this journey. I am eternally in awe of your teachings, practice, ethics, and helping spirit. You always know what to say and how to say it. It has been such an honor to learn from you, and I am beyond appreciative for all you do for the field of dance/movement therapy and beyond.

Thank you to the two people responsible for my presence in this world, my incredible parents, Richard and Susan Stockman. Words alone will never express all my gratitude, but nevertheless I'll try my best. Not only did you give me life, but you provided so many opportunities to me that paved the way for who I am and the work I do. To my mom, I thank you for your compassionate nature, never-ending support, and willing ear. I credit you for giving me my passion for helping others and my ability to listen. To my dad, thank you for instilling a sense of pride, strong work ethic, good sense of humor, and creative spirit. It is because of you two that I was able to write this book. You both gave me not only my ability to write what is on my mind but to express what is in my heart.

Thank you to my husband David, my rock, my best friend, and my partner in the business of life. Words alone will never express my gratitude, but I thank you for humoring all my ideas, supporting my every endeavor, instilling in me an entrepreneurial spirit, and cocreating a life I look forward to living every day. I cannot imagine this journey without you. You accept me, mind, body, and soul, and for that and so much more, I love you more than words could ever express.

Thank you to Sami and MJ for giving me an opportunity to grow and become more body aware every day. Being your mom has taught me more than I ever could have imagined. I am a better person because of you both. I love you to the Mars and back.

And lastly, thanks to you, the reader. Writing this book was a huge endeavor, with a mission that it spreads like wildfire—and that doesn't happen without you. Thank you for picking up this book, for believing in the power of movement, and for prioritizing your mental health. This book was birthed by me, but it grows and thrives because of you. Thank you for your attention and willingness to listen to my passion and purpose.

# Notes

## Preface and Introduction

1  Neha Christopher and Caroline Burek, "The Origins of DMT—Questioning the Western Presentation: A Reflective Discussion for Recent Graduates" (American Dance Therapy Association 55th Annual Conference, Dance/Movement Therapy: Creating Change through Global Exchange, New York, NY: The Association, 2020).

2  Admin, MemberClicks, "Home," American Dance Therapy Association, accessed August 14, 2021, www.adta.org.

3  ADTAorg, "Dance/Movement Therapy and Anxiety," YouTube video, August 28, 2016, www.youtube.com/watch?v=BnSKiPTJIDM&list=PLrbXrO8yG6hpvRWRnNTij7_CWTt2Th2J8&index=10.

4  Lori Gottlieb, *Maybe You Should Talk to Someone: A Therapist, Her Patients, Her Therapist, and Life's Essential Questions* (Boston: Houghton Mifflin Harcourt, 2019).

5  Dee Reynolds, Matthew Reason, and Bonnie Meekums, "Kinesthetic Empathy and Movement Metaphor in Dance Movement Psychotherapy," in *Kinesthetic Empathy in Creative and Cultural Practices* (Bristol, UK: Intellect, 2012), 51–66.

6  ADTAorg, "Kinesthetic Empathy: The Keystone of Dance/Movement Therapy," YouTube video, June 8, 2017, www.youtube.com/watch?v=a9uudFLSoP8&list=PLrbXrO8yG6hpvRWRnNTij7_CWTt2Th2J8&index=6&t=2s.

7  Peter Lovatt, *The Dance Cure: The Surprising Science to Being Smarter, Stronger, Happier* (New York: HarperOne, 2021).

8  *The Devil Wears Prada,* directed by David Frankel (Fox 2000 Pictures, 2006).

9  Aldous Huxley, *The Art of Seeing* (London: Chatto & Windus, 1943).

10  Bessel A. van der Kolk, *The Body Keeps the Score: Brain, Mind and Body in the Healing of Trauma* (New York: Penguin Books, 2015).

11  Lotte Veenstra, Iris K. Schneider, and Sander L. Koole, "Embodied Mood Regulation: The Impact of Body Posture on Mood Recovery, Negative Thoughts, and Mood-Congruent Recall," *Cognition and Emotion* 31, no. 7 (2016): 1361–76.

12  M. Häfner, "When Body and Mind Are Talking. Interoception Moderates Embodied Cognition," *Experimental Psychology* 60, no. 4 (2013): 255–9, https://doi.org/10.1027/1618-3169/a000194. PMID: 23548985.

13  Veenstra, Schneider, and Koole, "Embodied Mood Regulation."

14  Nan Zhao, Zhan Zhang, Yameng Wang, Jingying Wang, Baobin Li, Tingshao Zhu, Yuanyuan Xiang, "See Your Mental State from Your Walk: Recognizing Anxiety and Depression Through Kinect-Recorded Gait Data," *PloS ONE* 14, no. 5 (May 22, 2019), U.S. National Library of Medicine, accessed August 14, 2021, https://doi.org/10.1371/journal.pone.0216591.

## Chapter 1

1  Van der Kolk, *The Body Keeps the Score.*

2  Herbert Löllgen and Theodora Papadopoulou, "Updated Meta-Analysis of Prevention of Cardiovascular Mortality by Regular Physical Activity," *European Journal of Preventive Cardiology* 25, no. 17 (November 1, 2018): 1861–63.

3  Van der Kolk, *The Body Keeps the Score.*

4  R. Laban, *Choreutics* (Alton, UK: Dance Books Ltd., 2011).

5  Candace B. Pert, *Molecules of Emotion: The Science behind Mind-Body Medicine* (New York: Scribner, 2003).

6  "Dealing with Digital Distraction," American Psychological Association, August 10, 2018, accessed August 16, 2021, www.apa.org/news/press/releases/2018/08/digital-distraction.

7  Caroline Leaf, "Milkshake Multitasking," Vimeo video, June 14, 2016, 2:25, https://vimeo.com/170680229.

8  James Williams, "Technology Is Driving Us to Distraction," *The Guardian,* Guardian News and Media, May 27, 2018.

9  Van der Kolk, *The Body Keeps the Score,* 99.

10  Christine Caldwell, *Bodyfulness: Somatic Practices for Presence, Empowerment, and Waking Up in This Life* (Boston: Shambhala Publications Inc., 2018).

## Chapter 2

1 Caldwell, *Bodyfulness.*

2 Katy Bowman and Jillian Nicol, *Movement Matters: Essays on Movement Science, Movement Ecology and the Nature of Movement* (Sequim, WA: Propriometrics Press, 2016).

3 Katy Bowman, *Move Your DNA: Restore Your Health through Natural Movement* (Sequim, WA: Propriometrics Press, 2017).

4 John, "The Definition of Optimum Wellness," Coach Training EDU, May 3, 2018, www.coachtrainingedu.com/blog/the-definition-of-optimum-wellness.

5 Irmgard Bartenieff and Dori Lewis, *Body Movement: Coping with the Environment* (New York: Routledge, 2002).

6 "Laban Movement Analysis," LABAN/Bartenieff Institute of Movement Studies, accessed August 16, 2021, https://labaninstitute.org/about/laban-movement-analysis.

7 Peggy Hackney and Mary Konrad Weeks, *Making Connections: Total Body Integration through Bartenieff Fundamentals* (London: Routledge, 2020), 19.

8 Laura Cull and Juliet Chambers-Coe, "Rudolph Laban," in *The Routledge Companion to Performance Philosophy* (London: Routledge Taylor & Francis Group, 2020).

9 Nicole LePera, *How to Do the Work: Recognize Your Patterns, Heal from Your Past, and Create Your Self* (New York: Harper Wave, 2021).

## Chapter 3

1 Albert Mehrabian, *Silent Messages: Implicit Communication of Emotions and Attitudes,* 2d ed. (Belmont, CA: Wadsworth Pub. Co., 1980).

2 Martha Graham, *Martha Graham—Blood Memory: Autobiography* (London: Macmillan, 1992).

3 Marlene Jennings, "From Dis-Ease to Disease," Thrive Global, January 29, 2019.

4 Janet Barrow, "Is Body Language Universal?" ALTA Language Services, November 16, 2020.

5 Barrow, "Is Body Language Universal?"

6 "Psychology," Merriam-Webster online dictionary definition, accessed August 14, 2021, www.merriam-webster.com/dictionary/psychology.

## Chapter 4

1  Google definition, s.v. "Mind," www.google.com.

2  Hackney, *Making Connections,* 20.

3  Hackney.

4  Bonnie Bainbridge Cohen, *Sensing, Feeling, and Action: The Experiential Anatomy of Body-Mind Centering* (Northampton, MA: Contact Editions, 2021).

5  Crystal Jiang, Joyce T. de Armendi, and Beth A. Smith, "Immediate Effect of Positioning Devices on Infant Leg Movement Characteristics," *Pediatric Physical Therapy,* U.S. National Library of Medicine 28, no. 3 (Fall 2016): 304–310, www.ncbi.nlm.nih.gov/pmc/articles/PMC4922547.

6  "Walking Lessons—The Psoas Major in Infancy," *CoreWalking,* October 18, 2019, https://corewalking.com/walking-lessons-the-psoas-in-infancy.

7  Liz Koch, *The Psoas Book* (Felton, CA: Guinea Pig Publications, 2012).

8  Hackney, *Making Connections,* 16.

9  Hackney, 19.

10  Hackney, 42–43.

11  Hackney, 52.

12  Bainbridge Cohen, *Sensing, Feeling, and Action.*

13  Hackney, *Making Connections,* 67–83.

14  Hackney, 87.

15  Hackney, 108.

16  Hackney, 112.

17  Hackney, 119.

18  Hackney, 174.

19  Hackney, 173.

20  Hackney, 177.

21  Hackney, 198.

22  Amy Joy Casselberry Cuddy, *Presence: Bringing Your Boldest Self to Your Biggest Challenges* (New York: Little, Brown Spark, 2018).

23  Cuddy, *Presence.*

24  Helen Payne, Sabine C. Koch, Jennifer Frank Tantia, Thomas Fuchs, and Amber Gray, "Body as Voice: Restorative Dance/Movement Psychotherapy with Survivors of Relational Trauma," in *The Routledge International Handbook of Embodied Perspectives in Psychotherapy: Approaches from*

*Dance Movement and Body Psychotherapies* (London: Routledge Taylor & Francis Group, 2019), 147–60.

25  Payne et al., "Body as Voice," 147.

26  Hackney, *Making Connections*, 22.

27  Pert, *Molecules of Emotion.*

28  "Passing 4 Normal Podcast with Sharon Weil," Finding Ground in the Swirl with Amber Gray, SoundCloud, August 2020, https://soundcloud .com/sharon-weil/finding-ground-in-the-swirl-with-amber-gray.

29  "Passing 4 Normal Podcast with Sharon Weil."

30  Hackney, *Making Connections*, 22.

31  Bainbridge Cohen, *Sensing, Feeling, and Action*, 85.

32  Bainbridge Cohen, *Sensing, Feeling, and Action*, 85.

33  Daniel J. Siegel, *The Developing Mind: How Relationships and the Brain Interact to Shape Who We Are* (New York: Guilford Press, 2020), 17.

34  "Bottom-up vs. Top-down Processing," Khan Academy video, accessed August 17, 2021, www.khanacademy.org/test-prep /mcat/processing-the-environment/sensory-perception/v /bottom-up-versus-top-down-processing.

35  Victoria Rousay, "Bottom-up Processing," *Simply Psychology*, January 21, 2021, www.simplypsychology.org/bottom-up-processing.html.

36  Jennifer Frank Tantia, "Conversation about Private Practice," (lecture, Dance Therapy Advocates Summit), accessed June 2020, www .dancetherapysummit.com.

37  Tal Shafir, "Using Movement to Regulate Emotion: Neurophysiological Findings and Their Application in Psychotherapy," *Frontiers in Psychology*, January 1, 2021, U.S. National Library of Medicine, accessed January 1, 2021, www.frontiersin.org/articles/10.3389/fpsyg.2016.01451/full.

38  Shafir, "Using Movement to Regulate Emotion."

39  Dee Wagner, "Chi for Two® Offers a Piece of DMT," (lecture, Dance Therapy Advocates Summit), accessed June 2020, www .dancetherapysummit.com.

40  Hackney, *Making Connections*, 108.

41  Bainbridge Cohen, *Sensing, Feeling, and Action*, 104.

42  Tom Seymour, "What Is the Vagus Nerve?" *Medical News Today*, MediLexicon International, accessed August 28, 2021, www .medicalnewstoday.com/articles/318128#What-is-the-vagus-nerve.

## Chapter 5

1  Irmgard Bartenieff and Dori Lewis, *Body Movement: Coping with the Environment* (New York: Routledge, 2002).
2  Bartenieff and Lewis, *Body Movement.*
3  Bartenieff and Lewis.
4  Van der Kolk, *The Body Keeps the Score,* 27.
5  Bartenieff and Lewis, *Body Movement.*
6  Cuddy, *Presence,* 198.
7  Siegel, *The Developing Mind.*

## Chapter 6

1  Erna Caplow Lindner, "Dance as a Therapeutic Intervention for the Elderly," *Educational Gerontology* 8, no. 2 (1982): 167–174, https://doi .org/10.1080/0380127820080207.
2  Krister Nyström and Sonja Olin Lauritzen, "Expressive Bodies: Demented Persons' Communication in a Dance Therapy Context," *Health: An Interdisciplinary Journal for the Social Study of Health, Illness and Medicine* 9, no. 3 (2005): 297–317, https://doi.org/10.1177 /1363459305052902.
3  L. Palo-Bengtsson, B. Winblad, and S.-L. Ekman, "Social Dancing: A Way to Support Intellectual, Emotional and Motor Functions in Persons with Dementia," *Journal of Psychiatric and Mental Health Nursing* 5, no. 6 (1998): 545–54, https://doi.org/10.1046/j.1365-2850.1998.560545.x.
4  Liisa Palo-Bengtsson and Sirkka-Liisa Ekman, "Emotional Response to Social Dancing and Walks in Persons with Dementia," *American Journal of Alzheimer's Disease & Other Dementias* 17, no. 3 (2002): 149–53, https:// doi.org/10.1177/153331750201700308.
5  ADTAorg, "Dance/Movement Therapy and Dementia," YouTube video, April 29, 2014, www.youtube.com/watch?v=TYF9_zKDrc8.
6  Raed Mualem et al., "The Effect of Movement on Cognitive Performance," *Frontiers in Public Health,* Frontiers Media S.A., April 20, 2018, www.ncbi.nlm.nih.gov/pmc/articles/PMC5919946.
7  Van der Kolk, *The Body Keeps the Score,* 44.
8  Hackney, *Making Connections,* 177.
9  Hackney, 165.

10 Unibirmingham, "The Psychology of Rhythm and the Pleasure of Groove—Maria Witek," YouTube video, August 7, 2019, www.youtube.com/watch?v=Q9DyDMvAv2w.

11 About Paul G, "What Is a Native American Round Dance? History, Music, & Meaning," PowWows.com, February 26, 2020.

12 Wikipedia, s.v. "Haka," Wikimedia Foundation, accessed July 28, 2021, https://en.wikipedia.org/wiki/Haka.

13 "The Haka: 100% Pure New Zealand," The Haka, 100% Pure New Zealand, accessed August 16, 2021. www.newzealand.com/us/feature/haka.

14 Fran J. Levy, *Dance/Movement Therapy: A Healing Art* (Reston, VA: American Alliance for Health, Physical Education, Recreation and Dance, 1988).

15 Levy, *Dance/Movement Therapy.*

16 Gbenga Adebambo, "Movement Creates Motivation!" The Good Men Project, March 4, 2019, https://goodmenproject.com/guy-talk/movement-creates-motivation-cmtt.

17 ADTAorg, *Dance/Movement Therapy and Dementia.*

18 Jamie Marich and Christine Valters Paintner, *Dancing Mindfulness: A Creative Path to Healing & Transformation* (Woodstock, VT: SkyLight Paths Publishing, 2016).

19 Kittie Butcher, "Cognitive Development and Sensory Play," Michigan State University Extension, March 17, 2021, www.canr.msu.edu/news/cognitive_development_and_sensory_play.

20 Radicalartreview, "Rest as Resistance: A Guidebook to 24/7 Capitalism," Radical Art Review, September 11, 2019, www.radicalartreview.org/post/rest-as-resistance-a-guidebook-to-24-7-capitalism.

## Chapter 7

1 William Bridges and Susan Bridges, *Managing Transitions: Making the Most of Change* (Boston: DaCapo Lifelong Books, 2017).

2 Sharon Weil, Facebook photo, May 26, 2021, www.facebook.com/theagelessbody.

3 Erik Ceunen, Johan W.S. Vlayen, and Ilse Van Diest, "Frontiers in Psychology," *Frontiers in Psychology* 7, no. 743 (May 23, 2016), https://doi.org/10.3389/fpsyg.2016.00743; Charles Scott Sherrington, *The Integrative Action of the Nervous System* (London: Forgotten Books, 2015).

4   Amber E.L. Gray, "Polyvagal-Informed Dance/Movement Therapy for
    Trauma: A Global Perspective," *American Journal of Dance Therapy,* no. 39
    (April 12, 2017): 43–46, https://doi.org/10.1007/s10465-012-9136-8.

5   Fatina S. Hindi, "How Attention to Interoception Can Inform Dance/
    Movement Therapy," *American Journal of Dance Therapy,* no. 34 (November 14, 2012): 129–40, https://doi.org/10.1007/s10465-017-9254-4.

6   Maddie Burkitt, "Celebrate Earth: Be Inspired by 7 Nature-Loving Customs from around the World!" *1 Million Women* (blog), April 21, 2016,
    accessed August 20, 2021, www.1millionwomen.com.au/blog/celebrate
    -earth-7-nature-loving-customs-around-world.

7   "Celebrate Earth."

8   "Celebrate Earth."

9   Susan Bauer, "Body and Earth as One: Strengthening Our Connection
    to the Natural Source with Ecosomatics," *Conscious Dancer* (Spring
    2008), 2008.

10  Bauer, "Body and Earth as One."

11  Bauer.

12  Emilie Conrad, Continuum Movement, "CONTINUUM: An Introduction with Emilie Conrad," YouTube video, 2013, www.youtube.com
    /watch?v=IAacwbfveys.

13  Katie Asmus, "Embodied and Awake," November 10, 2020, *Katie
    Asmus on Nature as Healing,* Apple Podcasts, https://podcasts.apple
    .com/us/podcast/katie-asmus-on-nature-as-healer/id151987112
    7?i=1000498035127.

14  Sonya Renee Taylor, *The Body Is Not an Apology* (Oakland, CA: Berrett-
    Koehler Publishers, Inc., 2021).

15  Katie Bellamy, "Examining the Connection between Spirituality and
    Embodiment in Medical Education," Digital Commons @ Columbia
    College Chicago, accessed August 20, 2021, https://digitalcommons
    .colum.edu/theses_dmt/56.

16  Samantha A. Batt-Rawden et al., "Teaching Empathy to Medical
    Students," *Journal of the Association of American Medical Colleges* 88,
    no. 8 (August 2013): 1171–77, https://doi.org/doi: 10.1097/ACM
    .0b013e318299f3e3.

## Chapter 8

1   "Building Your Resilience," American Psychological Association, January 1, 2012, last updated February 1, 2020, www.apa.org/topics/resilience.

2   Lolly Daskal, "What the Most Resilient People Have in Common—Lolly Daskal: Leadership," Lolly Daskal, June 10, 2018, www.lollydaskal.com /leadership/what-the-most-resilient-people-have-in-common.

3   Eric Barker, "10 Ways to Boost Your Emotional Resilience, Backed by Research." *Time,* April 26, 2016, https://time.com/4306492/boost-emotional -resilience; Steven Southwick and Dennis Charney, *Resilience: The Science of Mastering Life's Greatest Challenges* (Cambridge: Cambridge University Press, 2012).

4   Kimberly Matheson, Ajani Asokumar, and Hymie Anisman, "Resilience: Safety in the Aftermath of Traumatic Stress Experiences," *Frontiers in Behavioral Neuroscience* 14 (December 21, 2020), https://doi.org/10.3389 /fnbeh.2020.596919.

5   Zab Maboungou, "Disruption Ceremony," (lecture, 2nd Annual Dance Therapy Advocates Summit [Virtual], 2021), www.dancetherapysummit .com.

6   Deepak Chopra, www.brainyquote.com/quotes/deepak_chopra_599933.

7   Conrad, Continuum Movement.

8   Doaa Kamaleldin Hassan, "Creativity Trilateral Dynamics: Playfulness, Mindfulness, and Improvisation," *Creativity Studies* 12, no. 1 (2019): 1–14, https://doi.org/10.3846/cs.2019.4313.

9   Lacy Alana, "Improv as a Healing Art: What Polyvagal Theory Teaches Us about Why Improv Works," *Yes And Brain,* May 18, 2020, https:// yesandbrain.com/blog/improvandpolyvagaltheory.

10  Hassan, "Creativity Trilateral Dynamics."

11  Hassan.

12  Levy, *Dance/Movement Therapy.*

13  Levy.

14  Lisa Fladager, "Mary Starks Whitehouse ... and Her Teachers," Movement in Depth, October 4, 2016, https://movementindepth.com/2016 /10/03/mary-starks-whitehouse-and-her-teachers.

15  Alana, "Improv as a Healing Art."

16  Patrick Bateson, "Playfulness and Creativity," *Current Biology,* Cell Press, January 5, 2015, www.sciencedirect.com/science/article/pii /S0960982214011245.

17  Dr. Arielle Schwartz, *The Post-Traumatic Growth Guidebook* (Eau Claire, WI: PESI Publishing & Media, 2020).

18  Pert, *Molecules of Emotion.*

## Conclusion

1  Caroline Leaf, *Cleaning up Your Mental Mess: 5 Simple, Scientifically Proven Steps to Reduce Anxiety, Stress, and Toxic Thinking (Grand Rapids, MI: Baker Books, 2021).*

# Additional Resources and Further Suggested Reading

Bauer, Susan. *The Embodied Teen: A Somatic Curriculum for Teaching Body-Mind Aware-ness, Kinesthetic Intelligence, and Social and Emotional Skills.* Berkeley, CA: North Atlantic Books, 2018.

Caldwell, Christine. *Getting Our Bodies Back: Recovery, Healing, and Transformation through Body-Centered Psychotherapy.* Boston: Shambhala, 1996.

Caldwell, Christine, and Lucia Bennett Leighton. *Oppression and the Body: Roots, Resistance, and Resolutions.* Berkeley, CA: North Atlantic Books, 2018.

Concepcion, Y. "Afro Puerto Rican Bomba and Afro-Dominican Slave Community Healing Approaches: Implications for DMT Theory and Practice." Unpublished master's thesis. New York: Pratt Institute, 2015.

Dana, Deb, and Stephen W. Porges. *Polyvagal Exercises for Safety and Connection: 50 Client-Centered Practices.* New York: W.W. Norton & Company, 2020.

Hendricks, Gay, and Kathlyn Hendricks. *The Moving Center: Exploring Movement Activities for the Classroom.* Englewood Cliffs, NJ: Prentice-Hall, 1983.

Herard-Marshall, N., and Rivera, M.E. "Embodied Resilience: Afro-Caribbean Dance as an Intervention for the Healing of Trauma in Dance Movement Therapy." February 1, 2019. Accessed August 29, 2021. www.criticalpedagogyartstherapies.com.

Magee, Rhonda V. and Jon Kabat-Zinn. *Inner Work of Racial Justice: Healing Ourselves and Transforming Our Communities through Mindfulness.* New York: TarcherPerigee, 2021.

Malchiodi, Cathy A. *Trauma and Expressive Arts Therapy: Brain, Body, and Imagination in the Healing Process.* New York: The Guilford Press, 2020.

Menakem, Resmaa. *My Grandmother's Hands: Healing Racial Trauma in Our Minds and Bodies.* London: Penguin Books, Ltd., n.d.

Nichols, Ebony. "Moving Blind Spots: Cultural Bias in the Movement Repertoire of Dance/Movement Therapists." Master's thesis. DigitalCommons@Lesley. May 18, 2019, accessed August 28, 2021. https://digitalcommons.lesley.edu /expressive_theses/150.

Porges, Stephen W. *The Pocket Guide to the Polyvagal Theory: The Transformative Power of Feeling Safe.* New York: W.W. Norton and Company, 2017.

Rivera, Mara. "Healing Aspects of Bomba: An Autoethnographic Study." Unpublished master's thesis. New York: Pratt Institute, 2008.

Stoner, Alyson. *Mind Body Pride: The 7-Step Guide for Deeper Inner Connection.* Kindle, 2021.

Whatley, Sarah, Rebecca Weber, Amanda Williamson, and Glenna Batson. *Dance, Somatics and Spiritualities: Contemporary Sacred Narratives.* Bristol, UK: Intellect, 2014.

## Websites

The American Dance Therapy Association
www.adta.org

American Music Therapy Association
www.musictherapy.org

Chicago Dance Therapy
www.chicagodancetherapy.com

Dance for Connection
https://danceforconnection.com

Dance Movement Therapy Association of Australasia Inc.
https://dtaa.org.au

Dance Movement Therapy Association in Canada
www.dmtac.org

Dance Therapy Advocates Summit
www.dancetherapysummit.com

European Association of Dance Movement Therapy
https://eadmt.com

Expressive Therapies Summit
https://summit.expressivemedia.org

Indian Association of Dance Movement Therapy
https://iadmt.org

Institute for Creative Mindfulness
www.instituteforcreativemindfulness.com

International Association for Creative Arts in Education and Therapy
www.iacaet.org

Kinections
www.kinections.com

Kint Institute
https://kintinstitute.org

Tamalpa Institute
www.tamalpa.org

Trauma Resources International
https://traumaresourcesinternational.org

## Body/Movement Practices

5Rhythms
www.5rhythms.com

Continuum Movement
https://continuummovement.com

Dancing Mindfulness
www.dancingmindfulness.com

Movement Genius
www.movementgenius.com

Open Floor International
https://openfloor.org

# Index

# About the Author

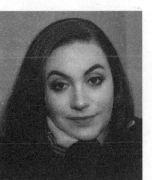

PHOTO BY RICHARD STOCKMAN

Erica Hornthal, a licensed clinical professional counselor and board-certified dance/movement therapist, is the CEO and founder of Chicago Dance Therapy. Since graduating with her MA in dance/movement therapy and counseling, Erica has worked with thousands of patients from age three to 107. Known as "The Therapist Who Moves You," Erica has truly changed the way people see movement with regard to mental health: moving people toward unlimited potential, greater awareness, and purpose by tapping into their innate body wisdom. In addition to her passion for working with cognitive and movement disorders, neurologic conditions, anxiety, depression, and trauma, she is an advocate for the field of dance/movement therapy. Erica created the Dance Therapy Advocates Summit in 2020 in order to spread awareness and inspire and connect individuals and practitioners from all over the world. She currently lives in the North Shore of Chicago with her husband, two kids, and two French Bulldogs.

## About North Atlantic Books

North Atlantic Books (NAB) is an independent, nonprofit publisher committed to a bold exploration of the relationships between mind, body, spirit, and nature. Founded in 1974, NAB aims to nurture a holistic view of the arts, sciences, humanities, and healing. To make a donation or to learn more about our books, authors, events, and newsletter, please visit www.northatlanticbooks.com.